The Fat Princess No More
A 107lb Weight Loss Success Story

The Fat Princess No More

A 107lb Weight Loss Success Story

Lori Lynn Wengle

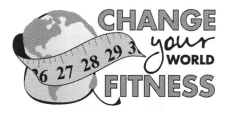

Howell, MI

iUniverse, Inc.
New York   Bloomington

The Fat Princess No More
A 107-Pound Success Story

iUniverse books may be ordered through booksellers or by contacting:

iUniverse
1663 Liberty Drive
Bloomington, IN 47403
www.iuniverse.com
1-800-Authors (1-800-288-4677)

ISBN: 978-1-4502-5285-0 (sc)
ISBN: 978-1-4502-5286-7 (hb)
ISBN: 978-1-4502-5287-4 (ebook)

Library of Congress Control Number: 2010912169

Printed in the United States of America

iUniverse rev. date: 08/11/2010

FOR EVERY PERSON IN THE WORLD THAT WAS EVER TEASED, STARED AT, TREATED LIKE A THIRD CLASS CITIZEN, ALL BECAUSE THEY DO NOT MATCH THE WEIGHT SOCIETY SAYS WE SHOULD BE AT!

FOR ALL THOSE READERS THAT SAY – "ENOUGH" – AND FIGHT BACK
KNOWING THAT GETTING HEALTHY IS NOT A NUMBER ON THE SCALE!

KEEP FIGHTING AND GET OUT THERE AND MOVE YOUR BODIES.

Acknowledgements

Many people have contributed to this book and I could have never completed this sometimes emotional book without all of their love and support!

To John Hall, my friend, colleague, editor and co-author for this book. Countless hours he spent fixing my grammar and telling me when I had huge holes in my story. I would write so much information and he would narrow it down for me, often confused, but he never gave up.

To my Mom, Marlene, who has told me over and over I could be anything I wanted. I believed her and did it, never thinking I would fail. And my Mom gave me another wonderful gift, my faith, often financially struggling to keep us in our Parochial school to ensure we had our faith deeply engrained in our life.

To my brothers, Mark and Greg whom I have always been close to and remain close to this day. They protected me growing up from bullies and teasing. Although sometimes the bullying and teasing came from them as siblings often do, their love and support when needed was always there.

To my father, Vince, who always wanted what was best for all of us. As a parent now, I see how much he wanted me to succeed and attain all of my goals.

To my family and friends over the years that always loved and supported me.

To my daughter Victoria, who taught me so much about my life, past and present. Although a young single parent when she was a baby, the joy she brought me PUSHED me to succeed and change my world!

And finally to my WONDERFUL husband Jeff, who saw ME! Jeff supported me emotionally while losing the last 60 pounds, always tried to help me finally be happy with my body and how I looked and taught me, it's really not about a number on a scale. Jeff bought me my gym membership and boy did that change my world. Jeff supported my goals and changed his way of life to meet my goals. And Jeff loved my daughter, who now refers to him as Dad. Jeff played Mr. Mom so many times, while I studied or worked late often helping Torri with homework, boy problems, life challenges, or anything that girl needed. And the three of us lived happily ever after....well Torri is a teenager, so as happily as one can be with a teenager in college:)

So many people helped me with this book and my product, including Spartan Printing, especially Jim Pierman, Shirley and Mark Lessner, Hub TV, Brent, Lindsay, Dawn, 10PoundGorilla.com, and my wonderful, inspirational clients that always kept going and kept me going!

John R. Hall

Co-author John R. Hall has been a journalist most of his life, beginning in elementary school where he 'published' a book of original poems. He graduated from Michigan State University with a B.A. in Journalism and has held several positions in the publishing and media trades over the past 25 years.

Hall is a prolific freelance writer, the author of thousands of business and feature articles. He hosts two websites where he routinely blogs and adds interesting "ideas." The websites are IdeaPerson.net and JoeMaintenance.com. He has also written three self-published books:

- Angels Working Overtime
- the NEXT Contractor
- Profit Tips 1.1.1.

Hall met Lori Wengle while writing a business feature about "Personal Trainer in a Box" for the local Howell (Mich.) newspaper. "The Fat Princess No More is a very self-revealing book which, while being cathartic for Lori, provides readers with a glimpse into the weight-loss struggles that are not uncommon for millions of people," he said.

Contents

Intro

I was an "average" child, if there is such a thing. In my early childhood the only thing out of the ordinary was an occasional temper tantrum when I couldn't have my way. But heck, we've all had a few quirks in our adolescence haven't we? The point is, I was just like many of you – happy, healthy, and "average."

Then things started to change a bit by the time I was six years old. I had become overweight. My Mom explained it away by saying the weight-gain culprit was actually a change in my daily routine. I had gone from the run-jump-play days of pre-school to the regimented world of full-time student, sitting in a desk all day and getting far less exercise in the process. Those three or four rolls of fat on my belly could be easily explained away. But it was not the norm. The sight of an overweight young girl was far less common back in the 70s compared to today, where obesity is on the rise.

The fact is, I was fat. And only a few other girls in my school had that same look. These were the alarming statistics:

- By age 12 I weighed more than 200 pounds and wore size 16 clothes.
- By age 18 my weight climbed to 225 pounds.
- By age 27 I reached 242 pounds.

I had spent nine years fluctuating between 180 and 242 pounds. On top of these ups and downs I had been battling high blood pressure – since I was 10 years old. My doctors explained it as hypertension (a medical condition where the blood pressure is chronically elevated) but I knew better. I simply thought it meant that I was too fat. On top of all of this, my blood sugar was also elevated. I was a mess and I was depressed.

I had to confront my mental and physical state of mind. At that point I was facing a very big decision. If I didn't so something about my weight problem I could become a diabetic or face serious health issues the rest of my life. On top of that, I couldn't even walk up the stairs without becoming winded. Exercise was the farthest thing from my mind.

Reality really struck home when I received a Mother's Day message from my daughter Torri, who was six at the time. As we all know, the wisdom of children goes way beyond their years – whether that wisdom is learned or unintentional. In this case, Torri had made me a beautiful Mother's Day booklet that described her impressions of me. On one page she wrote, "My Mom's favorite thing to do at home is rest." REST.

Now I knew that my weight was making a negative impression on my daughter, too. It was taking me away from doing physical activities and in a way, had become a selfish crutch to lean on. Torri deserved to have a Mom who was full of energy, not a couch potato. This was still another reason why I needed to CHANGE MY WORLD.

Around that same time (as if I needed any more motivation) I received the wedding pictures from my first marriage. (To clear up any confusion, Torri was born out of wedlock.) As I looked at the photographs I could not believe it was me. Or at least I was in denial over the true identity of the bride in those poses. My first impression was that the photographers were out to get me. Maybe it was an evil plot just to truly show how big and fat I was. It's amazing what photographers can do with lighting and later, with photo software.

My first marriage didn't last and I was hoping for the same thing with my weight. I knew that I deserved to be happy – both for myself and for the people I loved and cared about. And for me, it all started with being happy with the way I looked.

I had spent a young lifetime of being overweight or obese and being teased mercilessly at times because of it. I had endured terrible relationships with men and a less-than-fulfilling relationship with my own daughter. I was a single Mom who barely had the energy to come home and make dinner, let alone play with my daughter – a very great kid.

There was a really great person inside this fat body and now it was time to bring it out. I was convinced that it was time to lose weight and maintain it – to make me very happy and important. I knew I had a lot of great things going for me. I have always been a caring and loving person, a great Mom who loved her daughter and was smart, funny, and yes – very charming. But my weight held me back and caused much unhappiness. So it was time to fix my life – for good.

But setting a goal took a lot more than just losing a lot of pounds – believe me.

Over the next two-and-a-half years through lots of perseverance I lost and kept off 107 pounds. That sounds impressive. However, I did not lose the weight in the healthiest of ways. I often ate too few calories and the end result was that I wasn't a very pleasant person to be around – especially while I was dieting and trying to maintain my weight. In other words, I was a bitch almost all of the time.

And although I lost the weight I was very flabby and still tired all of the time. I just didn't get it. My body was saggy and I was still unhappy. On vacation I wore a bikini and my husband took a picture of me coming out of the water. To be blunt, I looked bad. My saddle bags and legs had so much cellulite and lumps; I couldn't stand to take a second look at the photograph.

Flash forward a bit. It took me three more years after the original weight loss to join a gym and then another ten months before I hired a personal trainer. Talk about a life-changing decision! Having a personal trainer helped me learn the proper technique, working each body part independently, and stretching. I began to see positive results very quickly. Fortunately, personal trainers know the importance of changing routines so the body is "tricked" and can never get used to the same routine. In my case, being tricked was a good thing.

For the next two years I weight trained regularly until the point where I was finally happy with my body. Yes, I "got my skinny!" Although I weighed the same as I had when I started the training, I looked 20 pounds lighter. Working with weights and learning about muscle confusion was the key. It changed my shape and finally brought out the true me. I was finally happy in my own skin.

Armed with a new body and a new attitude for helping other people who had experienced my misfortunes, I plunged into learning everything I could about fitness and nutrition. I took an online Personal Training & Nutrition Program and passed with flying colors. After that success I studied for the American Council on Exercise (A.C.E.) certification exam and passed it in November 2007. I had arrived.

To me, the phrase (and my business name) "Change Your World Fitness" is about becoming healthy, no matter what size you are. In fact, it has very little to do with size at all. What it really means is achieving your own personal best in mind, body, and spirit. I have changed my world and I would like to help you change yours. I know you can do it.

Chapter 1
In the Beginning...

Don't expect to read about the rags-to-riches girl who was discovered in a thatch basket floating down the St. Clair River after having been raised by a pack of wild animals, then thrust into humanity, by chance meeting a Prince Valiant, and then discovering the cure for cancer. No, mine was a fairly "normal" childhood, if such a thing even exists.

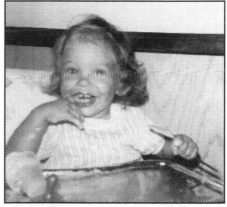

I was born on July 27, 1970, and lived in St. Clair Shores, Michigan throughout my childhood. St. Clair Shores is a northern suburb of Detroit. Its population was approximately 88,000 in 1970, a fairly large city. I lived in a neighborhood of ranch style homes on 60 foot wide lots and had many conservative, caring families in my neighborhood. I could see our family church and school from my front window. The city didn't really seem that big at the time. Maybe it was because of our close-knit neighborhood. Growing up in our neighborhood was fun with lots of kids and great neighbors that watched out for us.

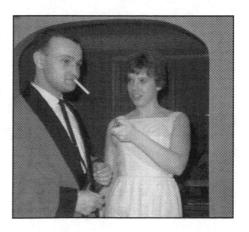

As for my family, Vince, my

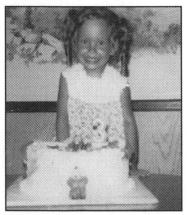

Dad, came from Malta when he was six. He had black hair and crystal blue eyes – a very handsome man. Marlene, my Mom, was a third generation Polish American, adorned with blonde hair and blue eyes. They met at a drive-in restaurant right after the death of President Kennedy and spent hours talking of the event. They married in 1965. My brother Greg was born in 1967 and brother Mark less than a year later in 1968. I was born in 1970 and was an "accident." Dad didn't want additional children, and Mom was on birth control. Unfortunately, no one was aware at the time that penicillin based drugs made birth control pills less effective – and I was conceived. An interesting note is my own daughter was born under similar circumstances.

My birth made the family complete – and I immediately became the apple of Dad's eye. My brothers teased me about it all the time, but I loved hanging out with Dad. I guess it is something about Dads and their little girls!

From a baby to five years old, I was a cutie and Dad was so proud of me. Being a girl had its advantages. After two boys, Dad was enthralled with his little girl.

Part of my charm was "learned" from imaginary friend, Tommy. Tommy was created because I really didn't have anyone my own age to play with until the time my best friend Sarah moved across the street from me when I was four-and-a-half. This lack of friends was especially hard on me during the cold, snowy Michigan winters when our time outdoors was

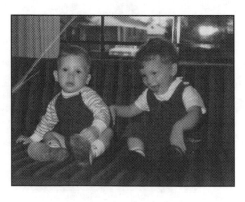

extremely limited. During those times if my brothers wouldn't play with me, I was out of luck. I think Tommy was created to make my brothers jealous as Tommy was solely "my friend," and I would not let either of them play with Tommy. One time, Mark said he saw Tommy. I asked him what color shirt he had on. Mark said red. In my mind, it was actually blue and I knew Mark could not see Tommy. I could keep myself occupied for hours playing with Tommy.

As I look back, Tommy could have been created because of Greg. He always loved babies and kids – and still does to this day. Greg interpreted my baby talk from the time I uttered so-called words. No one could understand my gibberish except Greg, and he would interpret to my parents and Mark. At four years of age, I began speech therapy, and became much more understandable. I now think there was never anything physically stopping me from speaking. I was spoiled by Greg's interpreting skills, and had no need to speak clearly. He always took care of us. Greg's nickname was "Mother Hen" and we continue to use it when referring to him, even today.

I would talk and play with Tommy for hours and Mom and Dad would just chuckle. One day we were driving in the car and I told my parents, "This is the house where Tommy lives." Dad parked his car and we started down the sidewalk together. Dad thought I would stop before we made it to the door, but not me. I was sure Tommy lived in that house. Once Dad realized I was going for the door, he scurried me back into the car, joking and laughing with Mom. I was teased about this event for a long time. In fact, to this day I'm still the butt of some spirited teasing from my family. Tommy lives!

As for my habits, eating was not at the top of the list. As a young child I was not a good eater, I really didn't like food very much, especially meat. But I would eat a Burger Chef hamburger once in a while. My other staples were fries, pizza, salad, cottage cheese, apple sauce, and desserts.

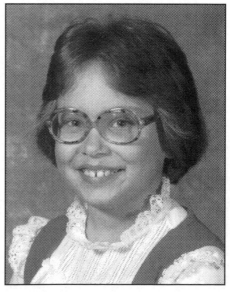

I had a dark side to me when it came to "food deception." I learned to stuff food I did not like into the creases of our snack-bar stools. One day Mom discovered my "cache" and I was busted. Mom or Dad wouldn't allow me to leave the kitchen snack bar until I finished all of my food. They would keep me at the table until I finished my dinner. But then Mom felt bad when I refused to eat and just sat there. She even brought out a purse-making kit to keep me busy. I actually wasted a whole evening staring at my food and slowly digesting it, which was immediately followed by my bedtime. Yuck.

And there was Dad, who would not let me leave until I cleaned my plate. I was as stubborn then as I am today, and I would not give in.

I just did not want to eat. But eventually pressure from my grandparents, aunts, uncles, and friends drove my parents to try using that famous and patented "Yucky Medicine" that my aunt used on my cousin. Mom says today, if she could go back, she would have left me alone, and would have just limited my desserts. I'm not sure if that would have worked either since I lived for desserts.

I'm not sure if these pressures to eat had anything to do with my years spent being obese or not but now I often wonder if it has a correlation. I certainly do not blame my parents. Now as a mother I understand how much we all want the best for our kids – and my parents were no different. I'm just not sure that best meant eating. In the 1970's life was different and I guess they just didn't know what to do with me. Oprah and Dr. Phil's advice was a couple of decades away. And in reality, I was a handful on many different levels.

Our educational upbringing was nothing unusual to write about. We attended parochial school, which was part of our Catholic church from kindergarten to 8th grade. We had two great neighbors that watched us before and after school while my parents worked.

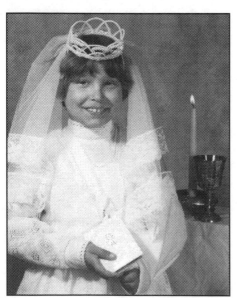

When not in school, we were a very active bunch. It seemed as if every kid in our neighborhood was out playing all summer long – from early morning until the street lights came on. At the time, I don't think we realized how fortunate we were. But looking back, we had some major fun. Between school and play, life was good – and at the time I thought it was "typical."

Speaking of typical, I was just

that. Physically, that is. I think I was a fairly normal size for a kindergartner. Mom even purchased size "slim" pants and jeans for me.

Then things changed.

Mom noticed it right away. She said that once I started full days of school in the first grade, I began to put on weight. And to add insult to injury, I also needed glasses! Double Whammy!

I was just bigger. It happened quicker than the other kids, especially the girls. I was a little taller, and much heavier. I was called fat for the very first time in the spring

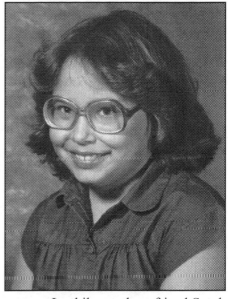

of first grade – and the taunt made me cry. Luckily, my best friend Sarah took me aside and made me feel better. She told me I was not fat. Her reassurance balanced all of the negativity in my six-year-old mind.

By the second grade, I had three or four rolls of fat on my stomach and was noticeably heavier than the other kids. Sarah and I made our First

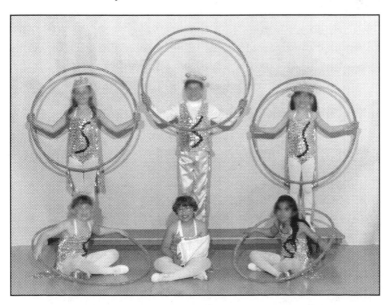

Communion together in second grade and the pictures of the event showed I definitely had a weight problem. The pictures show me standing next to my best friend. She was a twig and I was a heavy branch.

But my self-proclaimed obesity did not slow me down. In fact, I had broken my arm roller skating over uneven sidewalks and wound up with a heavy cast. Mom would even Saran Wrap and tape up my cast so I could "quasi-swim" in our pool, keeping my arm out of the water. When that cast finally came off, there were sticks, grass, leaves and all kinds of debris inside it. Nothing stopped me, extra weight and all.

I was probably thought of as obese by the end of first grade, and considering statistics, that wasn't hard to digest (no pun intended). For example, the average six-year-old weighed 50 pounds and I weighed 60. So I considered that obese. After all, 20 percent overweight is obese. I knew these numbers early – and often – in life.

During this time, I was being called fat on a weekly basis, either from my peers or my insensitive brothers. I knew I was heavier than the other kids, but I was still the fastest runner, the best jumper, roller-skater, biker, cart-wheeler, and anything I put my mind to. I became very competitive and had to be better at other things, to compensate for being fat.

One incident made me particularly proud and it happened around the time I had that dreaded – and lethal – cast on my arm. Teddy, a neighborhood kid was playing with me, my brothers, and some other kids in our yard. Teddy called me fat in front of my friends. That did it. I chased him and caught him and began beating him with my cast. He was three years older than me but that did not matter. He called me fat and I was going to make him pay for it. He finally began to cry. His Dad heard him crying and walked down the half block to our house, picked him up, and carried him home. I heard his Dad say, "You should not let a girl beat you up. Stop crying and being a baby. You are three years older than Lori."

Funny thing, Teddy never called me fat again. But, it marked the beginning of me being a bully to some of the kids. I would bully kids to feel important and good about myself. Again, a lot of what I did was a cover-up for how I felt about my appearance.

In third grade, I got a pair of Levi's jeans. They were from the women's department, size 27 waist. I loved them. I thought I looked so good in them and wore them all the time. But at that time, that size jeans were for teenagers and adults. At eight years of age, I was wearing clothes that were way too big for me.

Fortunately, there were some people who were sympathetic to my plight – namely teachers. In third grade, during fitness testing in gym class, I would wait in line with the other kids to climb up the rope or perform chin-ups (yes, I had a few chins, too). When it was my turn to perform, my teacher would have me go wait on the stage until the kids were done. It was embarrassing, but I was a relieved and somewhat happy to not to have to attempt something that was impossible due to my weight.

Because I was so embarrassed, I would either bully the other kids in class or use my sense of humor to entertain them, hopefully to make them forget what had just happened. Once back in class, I would imagine losing my weight, allowing me to climb to the top of that rope, ring that bell and receive an award. Right. Dream on Lori.

As I headed into fourth grade, things seemed to plateau out and my life went on as it had in previous years. But that was about to change – and Dad was in the center of it.

Dad was a workaholic, driven, hot tempered, held a grudge, perfectionist, etc. etc. But he loved me despite my "imperfection." He played tennis with me, swam with me, and I rode on the bar of his bike on many of our bike rides. At night I would sneak out of my room, jump over a crack that squeaked (Mom would bust me if she caught me out of my bedroom that late), and went out in the living room to lay on the floor with Dad and watch Johnny Carson. I still remember every episode and laughing with Dad. Even though the material that was too mature for me, I would begin laughing when Dad did and pretended to understand. It was a great time to bond.

I would sit by the heater in the bathroom and watch Dad shave in the morning before work. And I would be the first one to greet him when he came home. I would play and tease him and he would play and tease with me back. He was proud of me and made me feel loved.

Then, the bombshell.

In fourth grade Mom and Dad told us kids that they were going to get divorced and Dad planned to move to an apartment. I was devastated. Yet even at my young age, I understood. Dad did not treat Mom very well. And he did not treat my brother Mark well either. Although it was very hard and a sad time, I loved Mom and my brothers – and wanted them to be happy too. I missed Dad; but he would come and get me every weekend.

My parent's split did little to help my weight problem. In fact, it made it worse. I began to eat more, feeling the need to eat when I was sad or mad. That year was rough and when my parents fought over the phone or at our house it was very hard for me. They did the best they could in a bad

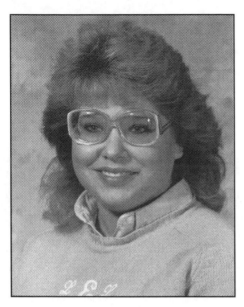

situation. Unfortunately this sadness had as much to do with me physically as it did mentally. This was the beginning of me "learning" to comfort myself with food.

And so now the table was set – literally. Between fourth and fifth grade I blossomed – or ballooned for lack of a better word. I went from fat to really fat. In fifth grade, I was wearing a size 13/14, the last size before having to go to specialty stores. And by the end of fifth grade, I had a huge safety pin keeping my skirt closed because the button would no longer reach the button hole. I was more than obese.

Even though I stayed in the same school system, I attended a different building of my Catholic school for sixth through eight grades. Up until now I hadn't given a lot of thought to having a boyfriend. And sure enough, by sixth grade, everyone had boyfriends. The quest for the opposite sex actually started for some girls in fourth grade but was really bad by sixth. The kids at school began attending our dances and naturally, bringing a boyfriend to the dance was the thing to do. Of course I did not have that option and felt left out of some activities. But fortunately, I still had a good time with my friends.

In sixth grade, I also joined track. I really wanted my letters on my school jacket and track seemed like the quickest and easiest way. My best friend Sarah and I joined together. During track practices that year, Sarah beat me in running. It was the very first time that had happened in our long childhood rivalry. Even though I was very big, I was strong and motivated. But my legs didn't get the message from my brain. I couldn't keep up with her any longer. I remember we were on one side of the field on a sidewalk and our coach had a stop watch. The first time, it was almost a tie – even Sarah was surprised. But after a couple of times through the line, Sarah was the true winner. My weight claimed another victim: running speed.

In our races, I came in last during every event at every school with every other track competitor. Did I mention the word every? But you know what? I received a standing ovation at almost every event I entered, because I never quit. Races weren't the only things I lost – pounds were, too. I lost 28 pounds over a couple of months during the track season. I was really starting to look good and even some of my cousins were telling me how good I looked. For the first time in years I felt great about my looks. So it was then and there that I decided I was going to run all summer – and be super skinny by seventh grade. I was going to get contact lenses to replace my very thick glasses and I was going to have a boyfriend in seventh grade and go to a dance in a fancy dress and be very, very, very popular. Did I also tell you I was a dreamer?

None of that happened. In fact I gained the 28 pounds back and 10-15 more that summer.

In fifth grade, I began menstruating. But due to my obesity, I had one or two periods and then not again until I lost some weight running track. Then once I gained the weight over the summer and I did not have period again until my 19th birthday!

Let me take a moment to explain. Many girls who are overweight or obese (women, too) are left infertile because of weight and other disorders such as PCOS (Poly Cystic Ovarian Syndrome), Endometriosis, Insulin Resistance and Metabolic X syndrome. I need a whole chapter to discuss this because these are vicious cycles and the only way to "cure" these is to lose the weight. There is no medicine to help. Physicians only prescribe other medicines to "mask" the symptoms, rather than help with curing the disease. Also, it was not until my daughter Torri was diagnosed that I realized how many conditions I too, had at that age. For girls having regular periods it is very important that they continue to be regular. Not having a period is cause for alarm. Upon going to my doctor, I was told I needed to lose weight to get my system back into order and if I didn't I may never have children.

All of the gains – both physically and mentally – in sixth grade were now a thing of the distant past. In seventh and eighth grades, I felt the worst out of all the first years of my life. I was obese, had thick glasses, frizzy hair, zits, a brown ring around my neck (insulin resistance), and was teased almost hourly. My brothers were at the high school and I had no one to protect me. I was a loner and shy, and it was especially noticeable when my best friend Sarah was not around or in my class.

The other girls all had boyfriends, so many of them were sexually active. I was definitely an outsider. Even though I still had a close circle of friends, I was sad and depressed. School was definitely getting me down.

Thank goodness for a good family and other adults (i.e. Mrs. Wilson) who inspired me to work hard and who gave me the knowledge that this was just a single point in my life. I had hope that one day I was going to lose the weight and all would be wonderful.

Before making the leap into high school, there would be another leap that would greatly affect my life, too. I decided (and was persuaded) to move in with Dad. Let me explain by giving a little "sibling" history.

I fought with my brother Mark a lot. In fact the last time we fought a hammer was used. Mark was physically and mentally abused by Dad. It was almost indescribable. Dad was so mean to Mark and it was apparent to me by the time I turned five years of age. I remember the first time, Mark called me fat. I cried to Dad, who lifted Mark up by his shirt against a wall and told him what a piece of shit he was.

Dad would not even look at Mark or play with him. Dad loved Greg and I but it appeared that he didn't even like Mark. As a result or as a way to "even the score," Mom began to treat Mark better than Greg and I. We even called Mark "Mommy's little boy." Growing up, Mark was into drugs and all kinds of bad things. Starting in middle school he hung out with thugs and was always in trouble with fighting and the police. But Mom protected him. When Mark and I fought – and I am talking knock-down drag-outs – Mom always took Mark's side.

I know that Mark needed Mom. She was the only one saving him and building him back up after a lifetime of physical and mental abuse. Mark never went with Greg and me when we visited Dad while he was living in his apartment. Only during holidays at my grandparent's house did they see each other. Despite all of the problems and fighting, Mark and Greg were my best friends. We spent a lot of time with each other as both our parents worked. It only took us moments to become friends after even the hardest and most physical fights.

But this last fight was crazy, and Mark was even crazier. So I left Mom's house in eighth grade. Dad bribed me to move in with him by promising to get me my first car at age 16, which he did. But of course, bribery should not have been the real motivation for getting his daughter back.

Chapter 2
High School Changes

A fresh beginning awaited me with new hopes, new boys and girls, and a chance to be popular. How? I was about to enter South Lake High School. I couldn't wait. And an added bonus was that this was a "normal" public school – meaning I didn't have to wear a uniform for the first time in eight years. My best friend, Sarah and I were going to own this school! (Or so we thought.)

On top of these already enormous pluses, my two brothers went to South Lake along with a few of my cousins. It was my turn to be cool and popular.

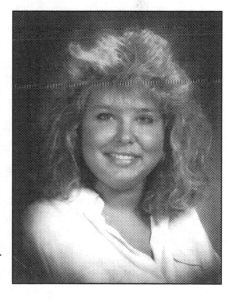

On orientation day, I woke up at 4:00 a.m. to start on my hair. Back in the 80s it took hours to do our "big hair." A can of hair spray and a blow dryer could make or break your day. The hair was complimented by electric blue mascara and eyeliner and a really cute outfit from Fashion Bug Plus. I was ready by 6:30 a.m. but now I had to wait until 10:00 a.m. That's right – hurry up and wait.

There was a lot of energy in the air at orientation day. I anticipated what a big deal being a high schooler might be – and that thought made the whole atmosphere more electric for me. In the end, it turned out to be less than anticipated. Sarah and I got our schedules and met up with a few other kids who were also making the jump from private to public school. It was exciting but uneventful. All in all, it was a good day with little foreboding of what was to come.

As the school year began, Mom, my aunt, a cousin, and I decided to join a gym. I went religiously with them. I was losing weight and got a new pair of parachute pants style that were denims. Finding jeans was tough. I spent a day trying to slip my butt into designer jeans like Jordache and Calvin Klein. But I still couldn't fit into any of them. I hadn't bought a new pair of jeans since the seventh grade, when I needed a pair for a trip to Washington D.C. And those were size 16 Gloria Vanderbilt's, which I eventually grew out of, relegating me to stretch pants or sweats.

Freshman year was difficult, but at least I liked the school better than where I came from. The cliques soon began to form and I went along with them – as stupid as they were – but I really didn't care. South Lake High was cool and the learning was a lot easier than my old parochial school.

I was teased a little, but I didn't let it bother me. Besides, my two big brothers were in the same school and if it ever got really bad, I would go to one or both of them and the teasing would cease. Greg was a senior and Mark was a junior. It came in handy to have two protective older brothers for a freshman sister. Even though my brothers did their own fair share of teasing me about my weight, they loved me and I knew they were just being dumb brothers to me. We exchanged a lot of spirited banter between us and I was able to give them a heaping of grief, too. So it all equaled out.

If you recall from my previous experiences, I never really had a boyfriend and wasn't interested in one, either. Ahhh, how high school has a way of changing perspectives. Sure enough, I developed a crush on Kevin, a football player. He was big and tall and funny. He used to tease me about throwing me in the garbage can. It was his way of being nice to me and he knew that I would not let him pick me up. I've had this thing against being picked up, even refusing to let my husband Jeff carry me over the threshold on our wedding night. I can't explain it – only know that I'd rather pick someone up using my own big muscles.

Anyway, I would tease Kevin about not picking me up – which was really a tease that blew up in my face, if you know what I mean. He was always kind to me and I think he liked me. But being kind was just another way of saying he really only liked me as a friend. Back in that day (and probably in most days), cute guys didn't date fat girls, unless they wanted to get a "reputation." But I always liked talking to him and he was nice boy. (You might want to hold on to that thought until you check out my 20-year reunion description to hear what he told me.)

As my high school years progressed, it seemed that my one-sided attraction to Kevin would be the closest I would ever get to any guy. I had a perfect record: no dances and no proms. I pretty much stuck to myself, except for those times when my core groups of friends helped me keep my head on straight and stay focused – and positive. We all did "normal" teenage girl stuff and had fun doing it. But that harmony didn't last forever. As we got older, all of my girlfriends spent more and more time with their boyfriends. So I did the most logical thing to me at the time: I got a part-time job.

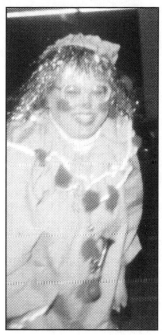

I became a bagger at Great Scott supermarket in Grosse Pointe Woods. Great Scott was a chain of stores in Michigan at the time and it was great to be making some spending money while trying a new venue to interact socially. At first I was shy, but then I started to come out of my shell. Sarah came to work there too, which really helped. It didn't hurt that there were a couple of cute guys who worked there. We all had a blast. I'm not sure why, but I was more comfortable hanging out with boys that I didn't go to school with. Heck, we even dressed up for Halloween and started hanging out together when we weren't working. I liked one of the guys, named Andy. In fact I had the biggest crush on him and he responded by flirting with me.

And then it happened. It is said that three is a crowd and that scenario is what drove a huge wedge between Sarah and me.

Over that summer, Sarah and I ended our friendship. Sarah had been pushing me away over silly things all summer while hanging out a lot with Andy. He gave her a tri-color gold necklace for her birthday – July 9th – and they were officially an "item." Sarah knew I liked Andy, but if we were no longer friends, then she felt she could date her best friend's crush without feeling too much guilt. Funny, I am now the Godmother to her daughter Jessica, so it all eventually worked out. As we entered our senior year at South Lake, Sarah and Andy were a couple. Looking back, the whole episode was heartbreaking. But we were 17 years old and this type of thing happened to me a lot. I had been dumped by friends as soon as they got boyfriends many, many times. If we were all to go back today, we would know better than to dump a friend over a boy. But we were just 17-year-old kids.

Truthfully, it really wasn't a surprise that Sarah and I were destined to split up. I had always been jealous of her skinny body. She was a beautiful Lebanese/Italian girl with a great figure. And I was, well, I was chubby Lori.

So, senior year started bad and remained bad. In fact, it sucked. I had no best friend and everyone else had boyfriends. I had no one to hang out with on the weekends so I worked as much as I could at the supermarket – and had one very lonely year. But I was determined to salvage something out of my years of loneliness in high school. I was determined to go to my senior prom. After all, isn't it every girl's dream to attend their senior prom? So during the spring of my senior year, I really tried to lose weight. Voila! I did – getting down to about 190 from 225. It also meant I could find some cute clothes in regular stores. I dressed to the nine's at the end of the year, trying to get a date for prom. But alas, my hard work did not pay off. Too bad. It has been in my DNA to work hard and I am always determined to get positive results from hard work. But I would get positive results later in life. For now, I was disappointed.

Like my whole senior year, prom night sucked. I sat home and ate. I envisioned everyone dancing and partying. I think some of my friends felt sorry for me or were just doing the "friendly" thing by inviting me to parties after the prom, but I was too depressed to go out. I felt everyone would be looking at me, saying, "She couldn't even get a date to her own prom." I was so down and out that I couldn't manage to go to school the following Monday. I didn't want to hear about how great of a time it was and I especially did not want to see anyone's photos.

Looking back at high school, many of the problems existed because of the obsessive way I felt about my weight. When a person feels bad about his or her body, their confidence is compromised. And despite doing everything I could to regain my confidence during high school – by going on "thousands" of diets and working out – I always gained the weight back.

I lived with Dad during my high school years and like me, he suffered through all of the ups and downs of my struggle to lose weight. He watched me become depressed – while devouring a ton of food. Dad felt bad for me, but he could not solve my problem. He tried to help me, but I was still a kid and would usually tell him what he wanted to hear. Predictably, I would never follow through. It didn't help my confidence when Dad reached his frustration with me during my senior year. By then he was disgusted with me and told me that I would never get a good guy – and that I may end up all alone. Thanks Dad.

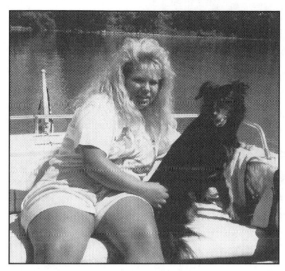

As Dad was berating me over my failure to keep a commitment to losing weight, he was forming a commitment of his own. He began dating a young girl, Pam, who had actually only graduated two years before me. Pam was not a vision of beauty – especially in my own eyes. She was – for lack of a better word – ugly. But she was skinny, which was obviously important to Dad and one more way to twist that knife that he stuck into my hurt feelings. He and I struggled for the first year of his relationship with "junior" and I soon took a step back – to the back burner of his life.

Our old times together, going to the tennis club, playing tennis, doing things together, became fewer and fewer. All of this happened at a time when I really needed Dad. It was my senior year and I was lonely; and now Dad had dumped me for his girlfriend. He promised to do things with me but it seemed that something always came up and Pam was right in the middle of it. On my 18th birthday, he promised to take me on his boat. He would be home around 10:00 a.m. but he forgot about me and went out with Pam instead. He did take me the next day with my Dog, Muffin.

Pam and Dad spent a lot of time together. Pam's parents knew about Dad but never met him, because of his age. Pam conveniently lied to her parents about his age. It took my brother Greg to break the news of Dad's real age to Pam's Dad, which sent Dad into orbit. Let's just say he didn't take the news well. Dad eventually married Pam in 1993, and he died in 1994. She did well for herself, getting almost everything that belonged to Dad, including his retirement income. Not bad for a 26-year-old woman. When Dad suffered a brain stem stroke in July 1994, she barely went to visit him until his death in October of that year. More on that later, for the present, things went from bad to worse.

One day, while fighting, Dad brought up my weight and he didn't stop there. He began picking apart Mom, too. That was all I could take. I believe that a Dad should have unconditional love for his child. Period. Not so for my Dad – or so it seemed on the surface. Fast forward to my own adulthood; I now understand that he did want the best for me, but he never learned from his family how to be supportive, loving, and accepting. My grandfather left my grandma for a time right after she spent six months in a cancer ward. She was 29, and came out with all white and gray hair. Dad had to raise his sisters and help out with the family, taking the place of his father. In reality, Dad's family today is all screwed up. They fight with each other and some of them have not spoken in 20 years.

Our family psychologist, Dr. Doyle said that out of all of us, Dad was the only one with psychological problems. We saw Dr. Doyle when Mom and Dad were going through their divorce. He thought all of us were doing well, but Dad needed help and didn't want to get any. Dad's life was not great growing up. In fact, he didn't have much of a childhood. So compared to his family, he treated me well. At the end, I knew he loved me and was sorry. But again, I was a stupid kid who was jealous of Dad spending less time with me. If I would have been skinny, I do believe he would have done more things with me and been proud of me. But at the end of his life, I knew he was sorry, I knew he loved me, and I knew he would have done things differently. I would have definitely done things differently, too. I was scarred by my "internal fight" of weight and obsession with food. I was in my little "high school" moment – thinking that my life was in the now, instead of the future as only a teenager could be.

For several years Dad had treated me badly about my weight. And now he was ripping Mom. I needed a change. I was an embarrassment to Dad. There were times when he wouldn't acknowledge me – even backing off from introducing me to his work colleagues. But he didn't hesitate to introduce his skinny nieces. In private and public he made comments about my weight to my aunts and to his friends, saying he didn't understand why I couldn't make a commitment and try to look better. My aunts were always telling me these things that he didn't want me to hear.

Although I do not blame him anymore, I remember eating more every time he brought up the subject. I remember feeling bad, sad, and angry with him over the weight issue. Dad had stopped becoming my support and someone to turn to. I was hurt.

It was time for a fresh start. I moved back in with Mom and enrolled in community college.

Chapter 3
Another 'Fresh' Restart

It was time to put the disappointment of high school and the rocky relationship with Dad behind me. A new way of life: living with Mom and getting a college education were probably the best changes I could make in my life. After all, the most important role model in my life both then and now, is Mom.

It was always important to Mom that I had all of the skills to succeed in life. She stressed the importance of going to college to all of us kids but the emphasis was even more important for me. She knew that I had to be college educated. With a college education, I, as a woman, could stand firmly and independently of anyone else. And she didn't want me to depend on a man to take care of me or to make me feel secure. This was an obvious backlash from her failed marriage to Dad.

After my parents divorced, Mom worked her tail off for the U.S. Department of Defense. She had moved to Virginia, working at both the Pentagon and Fort Belvoir, Virginia. Eventually, she moved again to Redstone Arsenal in Huntsville, Alabama. Mom did not complete her college courses, but rose to one of the highest civilian levels available without benefit of a college degree. She was admired by her peers, received awards, accolades, and was well respected.

She was a shining and guiding light in our family. My brothers and I were very proud of her and we always bragged about what she did for a living.

Mom told me early on that I could do anything I wanted. And I never questioned her. I truly believed that I could do anything I wanted. I never thought I would fail, mostly because Mom said I wouldn't. That is how much I believed in her. Failure was never a part of Mom's dialogue and therefore, it was never part of mine. Setbacks, yes – failures, no. It was no wonder that my plans included conquering the Earth and then retiring to enjoy the fruits of my labors.

If I could give any advice to women it would be this: Raise your daughters to be confident, loving, intelligent, hard-working, and always knowing in their hearts they we can do anything. And it didn't matter how much they weighed!

Speaking of weight, Mom had some of her own setbacks, too. Mom was a skinny teenager, or so I thought. But in the 1960's the girls were generally skinnier than she was. I thought she looked like a movie star, with the classic curvy body, and slightly larger than model physique. But despite my opinion, Mom had a problem with her own physical image.

According to Mom, Dad thought she had fat legs. But she showed me a picture of her after she had her second child and let me tell you, she was skinny. After Mark was born, Dad did not want any more kids. Maybe he didn't want Mom to get any bigger or he thought two kids were enough.

While on Penicillin for a cold, she got pregnant with me. Dad was already on a downward spiral – as far as his love for the family. His behavior was not normal, especially when he learned he would have a third child. Maybe his own personal family history was a foreboding of how he would treat all of us. And he was especially hard on Mom and Mark.

After my Mom had me, their marriage got worse. When I was six, my Mom went back to work in her Army civilian job at the Tank Automotive Command, where her career began.

Dad's anger toward Mom probably had a lot to do with her weight, although I never really saw that side of him until he began criticizing my weight while we lived together. He had a habit of keeping things from me, also known as his world famous "silent treatment." And he was the king of that. And he could remain silent for weeks or longer.

It wasn't just a woman's weight that bothered Dad either. After their divorce, Mom went on to a very successful career, which always bothered Dad. Mom was a superstar. Without completing her college degree she made it to one of the highest civilian levels of the Department of Defense. Every year she was receiving promotions and raises. She even purchased a brand new house. Dad was jealous. Although he moved up to running a drafting department at Michigan Consolidated Gas, the local utility, his temper held him back. His anger was not confined to his family, and he made his professional life miserable, too. When his boss retired, the company brought someone else in, instead of promoting Dad. I think it had everything to do with his temper. He stayed at that job until he died. He was a good provider, just not as good as Mom. She bought newly-constructed homes, traveled with her job, moved to new states, and had a great life. Dad always thought she would fail, but she tried even harder to show us kids that you can do anything if you worked hard. And she did it – in spite of her weight "issues." She proved that a person can be loved for who they are and not for how much they weighed.

Mom was our rock – and all of us kids were grateful. We knew she would always love us and support us. Mom also gave us our faith; something that I took for granted as a young person. It was not until I matured and had my own daughter that I understood how important faith is. The peace that faith can bring to any set of problems including my weight issues has allowed me to "let go, let God."

Being overweight consumed my entire life. It made me really irrational and depressed. Looking back, if I had spent the time working out and learning how to eat healthy instead of worrying what others thought of me, I would of "changed my world" so much sooner. But I was just a kid. Enough said.

Luckily, Mom kept me grounded, giving me the best gift any parent can give to their children: time and faith.

There was another great woman that I have to give a lot of credit for changing my life, too. Her name is Oprah Winfrey. Mom and I have been huge fans of Oprah since day one.

Oprah talked about her weight problems as far back as 1986. Like me, she went through a lot of battles – and a lot of hairstyles in the ensuing years. My hair and weight were a thing in constant flux. And at least I could share my changes with a popular television personality. Oprah was a good role model for me. She was beautiful, successful, and smart – all while battling a weight problem.

I loved her show and would watch it every day after high school and before work. It made me feel better to know someone else had the same problem as me and battled it. Oprah was proud of who she was and confident. She instilled a lot of that in me.

Mom and I often talked of her and we frequently watched her show together. Mom used Oprah as a constant reminder of how women could do anything, regardless of their size.

But Oprah and I were different in a lot of ways, besides the wealth and fame. She got skinny and I didn't. Once that happened I became a little self-conscious and didn't watch her TV show as much. I was proud of her, but I was not proud of how I couldn't exemplify her weight loss. But I was proud of my ambition.

Between my freshmen and sophomore years in college, my brother Greg and I worked a busy lawn service. We cut 65 lawns a week. On top of that I managed a movie theater at night. Talk about an ambitious woman!

I also lost a lot of weight – close to 50 pounds – and looked great by midsummer. I wore a bikini the first time in a long time. It was great. I went out with my friends and boys starting noticing me and liking me a lot. Even though I weighed 180 pounds, I worked out every day while cutting grass (the push mower way). I was firm all over and sported a golden tan.

I was feeling good about myself – for the time being.

Chapter 4
The Mike Debacle

In July of 1989 I met an older guy, a 26-year-old named Mike. I was not quite 19, yet quite ready for a boyfriend. He was cute and charming but a little too old, yet he became my first real boyfriend. I'm sure it was the attention he paid to me or the fact that I really wanted a steady guy. But he filled the bill.

He barely worked and lived in a house his parents owned, which was directly across the street from his parents. It seemed that this "freebie" was just one of the many things he mooched off of his parents during the years I spent with him.

About a year later, the life-changing event happened. I was pregnant. I didn't think I could ever have kids. Part of me thought maybe this was a lesson from God, telling me that I was very foolish and making a big mistake. It may have been, but I eventually got a beautiful daughter out of this. The fact is, I wanted a boyfriend or husband so bad, I would put up with this loser – and that was the mistake. It was all because I was fat and thought no one wanted me. So I was better off having a loser than no one.

The pregnancy was one event that I was really unprepared for. I had morning sickness for two-three months. I lost 20 pounds during my first trimester. I felt weak and could barely make it to work each day. And since Mike never worked, I needed to put food on the table and sometimes forced myself to go just to earn that paycheck.

I gave up my college education, felt miserable, and still managed to work; while Mike couldn't even manage to find a job – any job. I was the sole supporter. What made matters so ridiculously worse was that I had a new truck which I earned and paid for and he would drive it around all day while I was at work.

Fast forwarding a bit, Mike is still an absolute idiot. To this day he has no house, car, or job. He lives with women that take care of him. His parents eventually kicked him out for the last time, even though he has never supported himself fully. His Mom has enabled him from the day he was born. He has stolen from his parents, almost made his parents lose everything, and didn't care about anyone else but himself. Torri barely talks to him because of the way he treats his parents. She knows what a loser he is, not from me saying it, but from how he treats his parents who have done everything for him.

Yes, Mike was a jerk but somehow I managed to stay with him because he was the father of our child. In reality, I was about to be a young Mom and scared out of my mind. Here is a little insight: One day, while very pregnant, I drove him to a job interview. I was desperate for him to work. I walked in with him to ensure he actually filled out an application. It was a hot day and I was wearing short overalls with my huge belly sticking out. As we left the building, two girls drove up in a Jeep, looked at Mike drooling at them, and then called me a fat bitch. Mike laughed along with them and they drove off. He insisted that he didn't, but I didn't believe him. This was one of those "Ah ha" moments for me – understanding the true personality of the father of our child. Sure I was pregnant and fat, but I deserved better. However, I didn't realize it at the time and being pregnant only complicated things.

I could have sought shelter with Mom. I had made a mistake but Mom did not need for me to wreck her new life. After all she had done for us kids, at 21 I should have been able to do this on my own. But I was scared of not being a good Mom. Would I know what to do if my baby got sick?

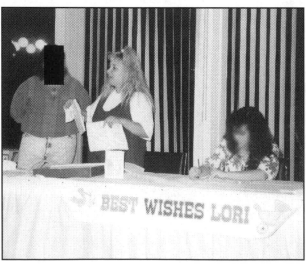

I needed that security blanket of having someone else around who could help me.

It was September 17, 1991, almost two weeks after my due date. I was sent to the hospital to be induced to labor. I was huge, uncomfortable, and scared. Actually, I was terrified. Although

21 years young, and smart, I just did not understand how this was going to work. I saw my private parts for 21 years and saw videos on the miracle of child birth but somehow I believed that this was not going to go well.

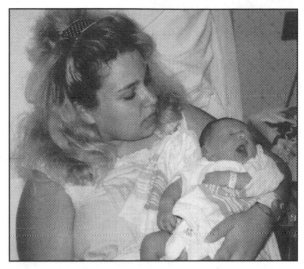

In 1991, having drugs while giving birth was frowned upon. I was going to do all of this with my breathing, not drugs. Once Petosin was administered at 5:30 a.m. to induce my labor, I started to have painful contractions almost immediately. My contractions started strong and came almost every 2-5 minutes for hours. By 5:30 that evening the doctor broke my water to try and help out with getting the show on the road. By 6:30, I was given something for pain, but it did not help at all. I could not get an epidural although I don't recall why. My problem was that I was not dilated past 3. I had to lie on one side because my blood pressure was going out of control.

By 1:30 the next morning, the doctor came in and asked me if I wanted to keep going or go for a C-Section. I went for a C-section. I finally got my precious epidural and all of the pain went away – in seconds. Thank goodness! I was scared and began to shiver. Mike didn't go into the operating room because he said he would have fainted. I was on my own. I didn't care – I just wanted Torri out of me.

The nurses brought Torri over to me. She was so little! (Or so I thought but eight pounds and seven ounces is not so little.) This was not like a doll, this was a baby, and I was her Mom. My family and friends eventually gathered in my room. After a few hours, I was fine for the moment, dealing with my new profession as a mother. But after they left, I was terrified. I never held small babies – never really babysat kids at all until they were two or so. I was so scared. I remember thinking the nurses might think I am a bad Mom and to not let me take Torri home. No one should have a baby at 21 – it's just too young. By then I knew Mike was never going to support either of us. His absence from the operating room should have been a good sign. The problem was, I was so scared to be a Mom and he made me feel less secure.

A day or two later, we went home. It was scary with Torri at home with us, but it was the best thing for me, to be alone with her. The following day, I had a hard, red arm and it began to hurt. When I first went into the hospital to have Torri, they tried to give me an IV. No one could find my veins and it took 21 tries to get a good vein, which was actually in between my fingers. It took seven nurses to find that damn vein. Well one of the spots they tried to put an IV in got a staff infection. I went to urgent care locally and the nurses told me to immediately go the same hospital that I had Torri at to seek treatment.

I went to the hospital and they were so nice to me, saying they would let Torri stay with me. Maybe they were trying to kiss my behind because of the IV problem. Funny, this time it didn't take them very long to find a vein – in my arm – and the IV worked.

I was not allowed to keep Torri with me because of hospital rules so I did what I feared the most – I let Mike take her home. Luckily, his Mom – "Nana" – watched Torri. Mike took my truck and drove Torri all over town to visit with everyone, except me. He barely came to see me and even the day he left with Torri to come and get me, he was four hours late – with no explanation for his tardiness.

After a few days of antibiotics through the IV, I finally got to go home. I missed my baby. I really enjoyed Torri. She slept through the night after the first night I came back home. She was such an easy baby to care for.

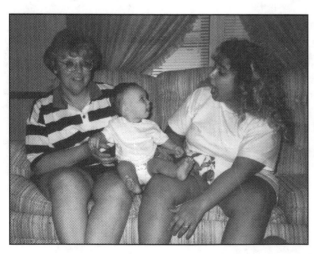

I felt the strongest love that I have ever felt for anyone. I had never been too emotional or cried easily, but that kid drove me to be a slobbering Mom at the drop of a pin. My life was consumed with everything she did. I loved her more than words can describe. Sadly, I knew Mike would never support us in any way, monetarily or emotionally. I felt bad that Torri may never have a good male role model, but I at least I would set a good example for her. Mike's parents were a big help, too.

And speaking of that slug, things went from bad to worse with Mike. He stole money from me while I was visiting Mom in Virginia. He cashed checks of mine and spent my car payment money. It turned out that he had been doing this for a while. I wound up three months behind in my car payments because every month I would give him the money to make the payment and every month he would say he sent it. But he would pocket the money. By the time Torri was born I was convinced that he would never support us.

One day, while working in the financial aid department of the local community college, I got a visit from a campus security guard. He asked me if I had a white Chevy S-10 pickup. I said yes. He described it exactly with my hot pink strips and graphics. He asked who would be driving it while I was working – because a crime was committed in it. I gave him Mike's name and address. Not only was Mike driving around in my truck killing time but he was also exposing himself to women – using my truck. What a wonderful example of what a father should not be.

I called his parents to let them know. Mike gave himself up to the campus security police. He left the keys and truck in the parking lot for me. That was the end of Mike and me. The torture was over. It's too bad I didn't use my own initiative to leave him rather than to wait for him to be thrown in jail.

When Torri was six months old, I moved with Mom to Virginia and then later to Alabama with her where I could finish college. I never told Mom anything about what Mike had done in my car. I didn't want to hear the lectures, disgust or the "I told you so's." She would not have done that, but I knew she would have been disappointed and angrier with him and his family. She was just pleased and thankful that I finally left him.

Mom never said too much about Mike. Maybe she figured the more she complained about our relationship the more I would rebel and continue to stay with him. In her wisdom she must have known that someday I would leave him anyway. She always supported me emotionally and assured me that she would always have a place with her, wherever she was.

Dad also got involved with the final chapter of mine and Mike's relationship. He picked up my truck from Mike and delivered it to the dealership. I decided to return it to the dealership because I could no longer afford it due to back payments and insurance issues. Mike did not pay my insurance or car payments. I still don't know where all my money for these things went, about $250 a month. I had bad credit for seven years because of this voluntary turn in, but it just had to be. I could not ask my parents to bail me out, so I chose to turn it in instead. Dad gave me a car to have while I finished up my degree. Maybe some guilt repayment? Being a Grandpa, he loved Torri. She was so cute and hard to resist. Torri looked like me when I was the apple of Dad's eye. I think that's what melted Dad's heart. Even my own Grandma saw the similarities and often called Torri by my name.

Although I could tell that Dad was upset with my decisions, he still loved me and supported me. It was hard for him to express to me how he felt. And he still had a problem with my weight. But he helped Torri and I out in time of need and that was what mattered most. He wanted to ensure that we both had a good quality of life. Dad's love never left – it just resurfaced after awhile.

IF I had never had a weight problems and IF I had enjoyed the "normal" times with boys throughout school I probably would have never dated Mike and Torri would have never been born, but I'm glad I got one beautiful thing – a daughter – out of the relationship. Mike was a loser. Period. During the first 15 years of Torri's life, I think the total of child support received was around $1500 dollars. What's that? A hundred bucks a year? Great. When Torri turned 15, we started to receive money from the State of Michigan. Was this some sort of mistake or a mysterious "gift?" I didn't know why the State of Michigan was sending me money. Our accountant investigated and discovered it was child support – from Mike. He finally got a job and was probably ordered to make payments in arrears. Thank God I never counted on that money from him but now it sure looked good.

Luckily the fruit fell very far from Mike's family tree. His parents were great to Torri and still are to this day. They have been embarrassed by him for years. In fact, he lived with them until a couple of years ago, well into his 40's. He made some poor choices.

On the other hand, growing up overweight and obese gives a person a whole different set of choices, including dating, jobs, and other important life decisions. I have to believe that deep down, a person facing these decisions probably feels that he or she doesn't deserve a good life – deep down. I know that sounds negative but that is how I felt about myself for a while. Call it a generality if you'd like. Maybe these people learn to settle and hope for the best. I learned I will never settle for less again, like I did with Mike. I also learned that settling for less has nothing to do with how much you weigh – it has everything to do with how you feel about yourself.

Back to life with Mom. I was only in Virginia with Mom for a short time – less than a year. While living in Virginia I was heavy – very heavy. I weighed around 235 pounds. I was depressed from the bad relationship, being a single Mom, feeling worthless, and very unhappy with my weight. But I didn't have to wait long to get a new attitude and outlook on life. Mom soon took a job at the Redstone Arsenal in Huntsville, Alabama. In anticipation of our move to a new life, Mom and I began dieting. By the time we moved I had dropped over 15 pounds and weighed about 220. I felt much better already and was getting my confidence back.

I enrolled in the University of Alabama in Huntsville in order to finish up my degree in accounting. I had to repeat some classes because some of my credits didn't transfer. But that wasn't a bad thing – I absolutely loved Alabama and the college. It was a great place to live and go to school. All the while I was in classes I also took step aerobics and ran for fitness.

Torri enrolled in "Kiddie College" and although it was a struggle at first, she began to love the classes and the other kids. Torri was so happy and that made me feel even better. I was losing weight, getting more energy, and climbing out of my depression. To top it all off, I was becoming a really good Mom, too.

Mom and I continued to lose weight the old fashioned way – manual labor. We worked our tails off on the weekends on her new house. I would cut the grass, she and I planted trees and flowerbeds, and we did a lot of activities to keep ourselves busy.

We tried every crazy diet under the sun, i.e. The Sugar Busters, Three Day Diet, and my favorite (although I can't remember its name). This "nameless" diet limited what I could eat during the day but at dinner, I could have whatever I wanted as long as I was done eating in less than an hour. An hour! Dinners were great. I cooked everything and had it ready when Mom arrived home from work. We had pretty healthy meals, but the desserts were a little naughty. We did lose weight because we did not get to snack during the day and after dinner we were so stuffed and content that snacking seemed out of the question.

I ran and rollerbladed on campus, often with Torri in her buggy. Along the way we fed the ducks in the ponds. I believe if everything would have continued on as it was I would have continued to lose weight and probably would have lived in Alabama for the rest of my life. I was even starting to get some looks from the guys at my school. Even though a lot of guys knew I was a single Mom (Torri and I hung out a lot together around campus) they liked me anyway.

And my confidence both from losing weight and excelling in college really made a difference. I honestly believe that I had the best professors, who helped me learn so much in the two years I was there. I was closing in on graduation, knowing the end was near.

Chapter 5
Losing My Dad

I took a light load of classes during the summer before my senior year in college. I was enjoying some of the beautiful weather and social life before getting down the nitty gritty of school again.

On July 8th, I was at a birthday party for one of Torri's friends, about 45 minutes from home. Mom was home and had received phone calls from an aunt and one of my brothers. I had a pager back in those days, but Mom did not want to alarm me.

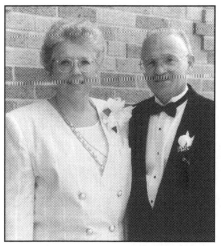

The news was bad. My father had suffered a stroke. He had been airlifted from his home to the University of Michigan Hospital.

When I arrived home, she told me the news. It sounded very bad and they did not know if he was going to survive. Later that day, we were told it was a brain stem stroke, which usually kills a person instantly. The prognosis of recovery was almost none.

Dad was 51 years old, always had his weight under control, very active, played tennis, and lived on a river where he spent the summers on his boat. He was a hard worker his whole life and was working in downtown Detroit at the time – an hour commute each way from home.

None of us could believe the news. He was seemingly fit and healthy – and not overweight at all. In fact, he was on the skinny side. But Dad did have high blood pressure and his hot temper and workaholic lifestyle did little to ease the symptom. At his job or at home, he was either working or sleeping in his chair. According to his wife, Pam, Dad had not been taking his blood pressure medicine.

Even though he looked to be healthy, in reality, he was not. Dad would eat at Coney Island restaurants, where he loved chili fries, hot dogs, and all kinds of other not-so-good-for-you stuff. He just had a high metabolism and good genetics that gave him a healthy look. But on top of not taking his medicine, he didn't like going to doctors. He often avoided them for as long as he could.

I wish I could have had the opportunity to teach Dad all that I know now about healthy living. I could have helped Dad get healthy on the inside. Maybe I would have seen his warning signs – but I just didn't know for sure.

Mom, Torri, and I drove to Michigan to see Dad and my brothers. When we got there, Greg, Mark, and Pam were waiting to fill me in before I went to see him. I was wearing my running shorts and a shirt. Both my brothers and Pam commented on how good I looked. In fact, they were shocked. I weighed 175, an all-time low since my days as an 11-year-old track athlete.

My brothers told me that Dad was on a ventilator. He would posture, which is when your body tenses up all the muscles, every 30 seconds or so. He could not move any limbs and could only blink his eyes. He was awake and alert at times, but because of the terrible pain in his head, the medical staff would drug him up a lot, causing him to drift in and out of consciousness. Greg went in to tell him I was here, hoping that we would not shock him too much.

When I walked in and went over to him, he sobbed uncontrollably. Nurses came in because his vitals must have changed dramatically – and they told me to leave for a minute while they calmed him down.

Even though we had some bad times, especially with my weight, I was still his little girl and that remained – no matter what. Plus, I was a size 13 and looked so much different than the last time he had seen me. I don't think he had ever seen me look better.

The next day, I visited again and we watched tennis together on television. He would look at me, unable to speak. I wish we could have talked because I felt he had a lot to say. I could only sense his sadness. Pam was in the room with us (one of her rare visits) while we watched tennis. One of the players was a young girl who looked overweight. I commented on how chubby she was and I could not believe she could play so well. She appeared to be the heaviest player I had ever seen on a national tour.

Hearing that, Dad began to sob uncontrollably again, and was posturing. Again, the nurses rushed in and kicked us out. It took a while to get him to calm down. Both Pam and I thought of what had happened and both believed that my calling that young girl chubby set him off.

I couldn't climb inside Dad's head but I believe that lying in the hospital bed, knowing his fate, gave him regrets to how he treated me about my weight. When I went back in, I told him, "It's okay Dad, I know you love me." I was trying to be strong and not upset him. But he couldn't respond to me – and I knew that upset him. Greg came in and calmed him down. I held his hand for a while until he fell back asleep.

Dad had wanted the best for all of us, but he was just a human being and made mistakes. He was hardest on Mark, being very harsh and inappropriate at times. Greg was not happy about Dad's marriage to Pam but they made amends. Dad was not happy about my weight and how it embarrassed him, but we got past that.

He was our Dad and we loved him and he loved us too. I know if he could've gone back right then to our childhood days, he would have made everything right. He would have spent more time with us kids and Mom – and they would have remained married. If Dad had a "do-over" we would have led very different lives.

And now, even though he could not speak, we were all able to make amends with him – including Mom. He wept with Mom as he tried to express his regrets and sorrow.

As a parent now I understand how important it is to want the very best for our children. Sometimes you have to let them fall, and sometimes you make mistakes, too. But you always love them. That is what I think Dad was feeling: some regrets, much love, and wishing he could turn back the clock.

Dad's prognosis was bad and his only form of communication remained his eye-blinks. He learned to blink his eyes once for yes and twice for no. Greg was there all the time, making sure Dad was cared for and that everything that could be done for him was done. Greg – and Pam for a while – kept everyone informed.

I returned to Alabama because I had to get back to classes. Greg kept me in the loop and gave me daily calls about Dad.

Eventually, Dad made the decision to be taken off the ventilator. He would never get any better and would likely have to live in a nursing home, dependent on a ventilator to keep him alive for the remainder of his life. To add to his situation, the nursing home he was at was apparently not taking good care of him at all. Dad had to be constantly evaluated to ensure this was exactly what his wishes were. He used an alphabet chart to communicate with Greg and stated, in so many words, that he didn't want to be a vegetable for the rest of his life.

I came back and said my goodbyes about a week before he was to be taken off the ventilator. Dad did not even want me there – and he told that to Greg. It was one communication he tried to make crystal clear.

While I said my last goodbye, I apologized to him for all the nasty things I had said to him as a kid, a teenager, and even an adult. I told him I loved him and that he was a very good Dad to me. I told him about all the great memories I had of sitting next to the heater in our bathroom watching him shave, how great he was to have the patience to teach me to play tennis, in which he spent most of the time going to fetch my balls from over the fence. I told him that the laughter we shared watching Johnny Carson was my favorite memory – and that our "alone time" meant a lot to me.

I told Dad that I understood his disappointment in my weight and my bad decisions. But I was going to make him really proud of me, even if he was watching from Heaven. I asked him to keep an eye on Torri from Heaven – and he cried.

I thought I would spend the day with him, but 20 minutes was all we both could take. I did not go back the next day as Greg told me that my visit had been very hard on Dad emotionally. I flew home and waited for the call when they had removed the ventilator. Greg was with him every day to ensure this is what he wanted. When he asked Dad, the response was a yes eye-blink every time. Greg even videotaped Dad giving his permission to be removed from the ventilator, ensuring that his wishes were fully understood and documented.

On the day he was to be removed from the ventilator, the doctors gave Dad some medicine to make sure he could relax. They wanted to make sure he was "out of it" a little as he would not be able to breathe. Greg said that when they got closer to removing the ventilator, Dad's eyes got big, waiting for death. When they removed the ventilator, Dad started to breath on his own. No one could believe it.

But because he was never going to recover, Dad asked for his feeding tube to be removed. Six weeks later on October 29th, Dad finally was at peace. The man I loved and fought with all of my life had passed away.

Mom, Torri, and I came back up for my Dad's funeral. Many people from his work, our neighborhood, friends, and family attended. Our family pulled together and remembered the really good times – because there really were so many good times.

I just wish there would have been more time to experience more of the good times. I wish Dad could still be with us to see all of us as we are now. And just as importantly, I wish Dad could be with our family during holidays, birthdays, Father's Day – let's just say any day.

I have a very long "wish list" now. I wish I could have taught Dad to eat healthy, exercise often, and to lead a healthy life. I wish Dad would know me now all grown up and responsible. I wish Dad could see me in "my skinny" as a fitness instructor. I wish Dad could see me and know me now.

Chapter 6
The Tom Years

While at Dad's funeral, I was reintroduced to Greg's best friend, Tom. He was hilariously funny – even cracking us up at the funeral. It was a very solemn and sad time for us after the burial – the finality had become reality. Yet Tom kept us distracted, keeping us in tears of laughter instead of sorrow. He was exactly what we all needed.

Tom had been Greg's friend since freshman year in high school. When Tom would come over to visit Greg, I would answer the door and see who it was. Once I saw it was Tom I slammed the door in his face and went and sat down. I did not like Tom. I thought he was rude, crude, and hairy.

As strange as it may seem, Dad's wife Pam was supposed to go to the prom with Tom back in high school. The day of the prom, Tom stood her up. As I said before, Pam was skinny, but really unattractive and even unattractive to Tom, eventually making him see the light before taking her to the prom. He told me her bad acne made him want to throw up. I loved hearing that because by then I couldn't stand Pam. When Dad and Pam eventually got together, I could not stand her, and then she tried to befriend me knowing she could spend more time with Dad if she was nice to me. I hated her because of her manipulative ways. But I digress.

After the funeral I began to talk to Tom on the phone and went over to his new house before I left for school again in Alabama. A few months later during Christmas I was back in Michigan. Tom came to my aunt's house with me to celebrate and attended mass with my family.

Tom was so funny; people could not help but like him. He had a sense of humor like my brothers and said very off-the-wall comments. We had a fun time, and I laughed and laughed and laughed at his humor. In the beginning even four-year-old Torri liked him.

We "dated" over the phone for the next six months. At about that time I decided it was best to move back to Michigan to be near my family – and

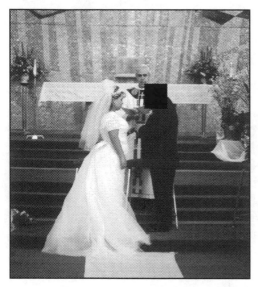

Tom. Fortunately I inherited a small amount of money, got a job, and finished up my degree at night over the next year.

I missed my brothers, Tom, and my cousins. Mom seemed to be working a lot for Redstone Arsenal. She was not happy with Tom at all and thought I could do better. She didn't like his crudeness or the way he joked about Torri. Mom didn't like his sense of humor either.

I was lonely and not quite sure why I wanted to date and later marry Tom. I know if Dad hadn't been hospitalized, I would have never even dated Tom. But losing my father made me want a family. I weighed 175 pounds and was confident, graduating Magna Cum Laude from college. But I still wanted a family. I wanted to be loved.

And then it happened. Tom popped the question. We got engaged and he bought me a huge engagement ring. It seemed like the right thing to do – and it felt right.

Tom had his own business, which brought with it all of the problems of ownership including clashing personalities and managing a budget. He usually spent more than he earned and soon, my job and inheritance was

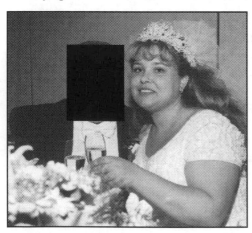

paying for more "stuff" including our huge Italian wedding and home remodeling.

Ah yes, we had our big wedding. Looking back now, it is easy to say everything in my life changed after that night – and not all for the good. The wedding was beautiful, probably because I spent a fortune on it. I had a beautiful slim style dress on my chunky frame. Why? Because I had gained all the weight I lost and then some. I'll explain in a moment.

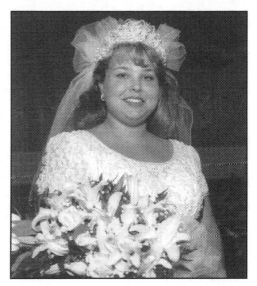

On my wedding day I weighed 242 pounds. Since ordering the dress I had gained 25 of those pounds and at my last fitting, the woman said that if I gained any more weight, the dress would not fit me. Being in denial, I thought she ordered it too small anyway. But no, she showed me the measurements and I really had gained all of that weight. She let out as much as she could, but it was still very tight. This added to my already tense life right before the wedding.

I had to wear two girdles to fit into the too-tight dress. At the time, I really thought I looked wonderful. I tried so hard but my weight had come back to haunt me. Even at the last minute from the back of church, some of the women were helping me, trying to pull down my short sleeves to hide a lump of fat on the back of my arms. The sleeves were so tight, this lump kept coming out, and even as I was walking down the aisle, they were adjusting me.

In case you have not gotten it yet, I eat when I am sad, mad, or unhappy. This was a time in my life for sadness because in retrospect, I never should have married Tom. I knew it and my family knew it. I just wanted to be loved and have a normal family like everyone else. I wanted a husband and father for my daughter. I wanted to be a wife, albeit a fat wife. So I settled for Tom, again, thinking I did not deserve a cute, educated person.

To be blunt, Tom stopped being a gentleman. Even on our honeymoon he was rude, ordering me to grab my own luggage. Everything was different. He was not as nice to me or Torri. Saying "I do" translated into "I don't have to be nice any more."

About six weeks after the wedding I got my much-anticipated wedding album. I was horrified. I paid $1,800 for my photographers and album and what did I get? More bad news. All the pictures were horrible. I was convinced my photographers were out to get me. They took pictures to make me look fat, or so I reasoned. The pictures looked nothing like me. But

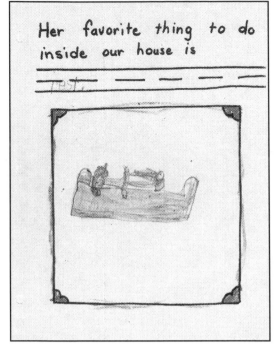

Her favorite thing to do inside our house is

Tom, standing right next to me, looked normal, like himself. I rationalized that something was amiss. I never even ordered my wedding album and the photographers would not give me any sort of refund.

The next week was Mothers Day at Torri's school. She was in first grade at St. Joan of Arc. I was so excited when Torri told me how hard she was working on a present for me and that night, she would get to give it to me in front of her class. I knew a little bit, because she was asking me questions that I thought would translate into a book about my life.

That evening I went to the event in Torri's classroom. I sat at those little first grade chairs. Actually I had two little chairs, one for each cheek, so to speak. It was Torri's turn to read her book about her Mom. She was not nervous. I thought she may be with all the parents around and with her shyness and all. Torri was pumped up, knowing that I would love this present.

She began reading her book titled "All about Mom." It was so cute and Torri was so enthusiastic as she read it, showing the pictures. She drew great pictures of me with my big, frizzy hair. It was outstanding. Finally, near the end of the book, Torri read, "My Mom's favorite thing to do inside our house: REST!" With that caption went a picture of me sprawled out on our couch watching TV. I could feel the heat start at my feet and work up to my head. I was embarrassed as were all the other "good parents" who were looking at me. And even though I was smiling at Torri, she knew it was not good. She did not finish reading her book, choosing instead to run over to me and put her head in my arm. I tried to console her as she meant to please me – and not make me sad.

On the way home, we talked, and I said to her, "Mommy is not mad at you, Mommy is mad at herself. Mommy gained weight, was unhappy, and was so tired after work every day." It was right then that I promised myself, no more. I was not going to gain any more weight. In fact I was going to lose weight. Torri deserved a Mom who had energy to play with her and not lay on the couch every night. I said, "That's it, I have had enough."

I began to lose weight, using not the healthiest ways: diet pills, Diet Coke and cigarettes. It wasn't exactly doctor recommended. But I was going to lose the weight for good. I was going to be a good, in-shape Mom and that was it. Before long, I began to stick up for myself and my daughter more and more against Tom. We began to spend more time apart from Tom, visiting my brothers more.

That was good, because for a while, Tom had been treating Torri and me differently. At times, I had to step in and ask him not to yell at Torri or call her names. She was my child, not his. Plus she was only a five-year-old who had already been through a lot of tough life changes.

Tom was not all bad. The three of us had a lot of good times. But the bad times kept multiplying – and his hot Italian temper was showing itself more and more. His father had parented him the same way he wanted to father Torri – by doing a lot of yelling. But I already experienced enough yelling from my own father, and did not want it for Torri.

One day, at a family baby or bridal shower (I can't remember which), my cousin and aunt from Mom's side of the family told my cousins and aunts on Dad's side of the family that Tom shoved Torri and was mean to her in their presence. At first I was very mad at my family for gossiping – which they were very good at. Somehow bashing us behind our backs had become normal. But I was glad they spoke up.

I saw Tom's changes and I didn't like them at all. It was easy to see why I gained all of my weight back plus more before our wedding. The changes had happened long before the "I do's."

Both my brothers counseled me. They had seen Tom's treatment of me and Torri and didn't like it. Greg, still his best friend to this day, told me that Tom was going to be like his Dad and he was never going to change. I knew Tom's childhood story and how his Dad was. Knowing he wouldn't change was an unnerving thought.

Luckily, I relied on my family again. Mark took Torri and me in on the weekends. Because Torri was in school, her Nana and Papa (Mike's parents) took her during the week. Torri still had six months to go to finish second grade.

While still married to Tom, I got a great job at Nextel Communications. So I was already making a great living. Now it was time to break the ties and get rid of that ball-and-chain named Tom. Soon after I got a new promotion at Nextel I filed for divorce and went on with my life. I lost about 50 pounds and was feeling pretty good.

My plans involved moving away from the old neighborhood and getting closer to where I worked. I wanted to find a place in Brighton, where I wanted to live. I really liked the rural atmosphere, which I fell in love with. I became acquainted with the homes in the area by reading a lot of real estate books.

I was determined to buy a house, get Torri enrolled in school for the next year, and be alone – possibly to never date again. I really sucked with men and thought time alone would be great for Torri and me. I was almost to the point of hating men and began to male bash at work. That was okay, because I was on my way to the top of my profession. I climbed the corporate ladder, became a top senior dealer manager for Nextel, and was making enough money to support Torri and myself. I had lost 50 pounds and was down to 195, only 15 pounds away from my "normal skinny" of 180.

I was never going to be overweight, take any man's crap, need any man – none of that. I was going to be a Mom, and an energetic Mom at that.

Chapter 7
Free at Last

I was starting a new chapter in my life now that I was free of Tom and a little less stressed out from the previous tumultuous years. So naturally I was feeling good about things, which meant I was happy and eating less. I was determined more than ever to lose weight and keep it off. But I went about it the wrong way,

I literally starved myself for two years, living on diet pills, Diet Coke and cigarettes to lose weight. There's nothing like putting a lot of bad things into my body. And I would eat as few as 300-500 calories a day. Overall, that's a pretty whacked-out diet and one that I would never ever recommend.

As you have read up until now, I had been very unhappy as an over-weight child, teen, and adult. The biggest struggle in my life was my weight – and I was obsessed with it.

I have been on every diet under the sun. You name it, I have done it. I read about every diet in every magazine and tried it. I read every advertisement for every product in every magazine. I tried every diet book, every celebrity diets, and followed Oprah Winfrey's diet. I have taken Phen Phen, Metabolife with Ephedrine, Hydroxcut – everything. Want more? I tried a cabbage soup diet (complete with a healthy supply of odorous gas afterward), a three-day diet that was developed for overweight people before surgery, the sugar busters diet, the eat-anything-you-want-at-dinner diet (had another name, but not sure), and the grapefruit diet. I did deal-a-meal by Richard Simmons (which is actually a very balanced easy-to-use diet that I still really like), the Medical Weight Loss Clinics, LA Weight Loss, Weight Watchers, etc. But I never kept the weight off.

I have spent so much money on all these diets. I joke that if I had all the money I spent on losing weight; I could have paid for my daughter's college education at the very least and maybe thrown in a new car for myself as well.

I was so desperate to break the cycle and change my world for Torri and me. During the time I was leaving Tom, I did lose 40-50 pounds and was feeling really good about myself. Even Torri was telling me how pretty and skinny I was. She could get her tiny little arms around my waist now, just barely.

I had thrown myself into my work at Nextel. I was on the road five days a week, but I refused to eat roadie food. So I would pack some celery sticks and Diet Coke in a cooler. That is all I ate all day. Yes, I was hungry, but the Metabolife with Ephendra took care of my hunger pains and day after day, I would continue on with it. At night I would eat cottage cheese and ten grapes (not eleven) and go to bed.

I excelled at Nextel, won tons of awards, cash bonuses, and five star vacations to all kinds of great places. But the success didn't alter my eating habits. I kept on dieting.

It wasn't all good. The dieting took its toll on my body. I began to have dizzy spells, low blood pressure, low sugar, and believe it or not, my hair began to fall out. I was tired and crabby at home and felt terrible. If this was the downside to dieting I wondered if there was any upside (besides shedding pounds).

But I kept starving myself. I would set a goal, which included the following statement, "Oh if I could only weigh this much on the scale, then I would be happy." Problem was, I would achieve that goal and still not be happy. Then I would set another goal, and again once I achieved it, and was still not be happy.

The compliments on my new look were coming from everywhere. Men were staring and paying more attention to me. They were holding the doors for me. Men asked for my phone number. I was on the road in my car and a lot of truckers would honk at me – and it wasn't because I was driving erratically. They liked what they saw in the front seat. I loved feeling attractive and finally somewhat normal sized. But I was still unhappy with my body.

I was probably a combination of crazy and obsessed by then. I starved and starved for two years and finally weighed 135 pounds. In clothes I looked good, but out of clothes or in a swimsuit, I wasn't happy. Was there any happy medium?

I was hungry, crabby, tired, dizzy, and sometimes felt like I would never be happy with my body and body image. Even at 135 pounds, I was still seeing that fat Lori. Something had to give.

I was very self-conscious, too. If a thin girl walked into the room, I began to multiply in size, letting my mind add pounds to my frame. If a woman my own size came into the room, my mind would tell me that I was still bigger and fatter than her.

My dizzy spells got worse and I ended up blacking out several times. After one blackout, my doctor told me to go to the hospital emergency room. Because of all the crap I put into my body, especially diet pills, I had a low blood pressure problem. And I would not eat anything with sodium. I failed a "tilt table" test, which is an indication of this type of problem. My prescription was to make sure I was fully hydrated and eating some salt. Even now I carry water and pretzels in my purse every day, just in case I feel faint. I know how to read my body signals and I don't need any more emergency room visits or wake-up calls.

So let's recap. Diets don't work. And another thing – don't get on a diet and stay on it for the rest of your life. Take it from someone who knows, this type of behavior or lifestyle is not good for you nor will it effectively help you lose weight. I know now that eating healthy, from all the food groups is what my body needs. And most importantly, exercise will make the biggest difference in your body image.

Here's a little secret tidbit for all the women and men out there. Do you know that when skinny girls tell you they are fat, they really mean it? They do, no kidding. Until I thinned down I wouldn't believe it if I heard it. Here I was, a big fat thing and a skinny little girl would claim she was fat. I wanted to slap those little bodies all over the place. Let's face it – all girls are crazy, whether they are skinny or overweight – men, too. Exercise will reduce or eliminate some of this craziness because feeling fit gives anybody a whole new perspective on life – and much more self confidence. Exercise will make you happy with the way you look. (If you think this is a perfect segue into rest of the book, you are correct.)

So, once again, let's do another recap. Diets do not work. If a diet is void of fruit, it is not a good diet. If a diet cuts pizza out of your routine, it is not a good diet. If a diet frowns on wine consumption, throw that one away. If a diet excludes red meat, don't give it a second thought.

Try eating healthy, better complex carbs, lean meats, low fat dairy, lots of green veggies, lots of veggies in general, a couple fruits a day, and drink lots of water. You can't go wrong with these ingredients.

Eating healthy is what our bodies require; they run like a well tuned machine to help us get through our crazy lives. When I eat something "bad" such as greasy foods, I feel terrible for days; my body does not want that. It wants complex carbs, lean meats and good foods.

Okay, I'll get off my soapbox for now. On with my story. During the time of diet changes and general bodily upheaval, I began a relationship with a man that CHANGED MY WORLD for the better – finally. I found a really good man whom I love and adore to this very day. I had never felt this kind of love. And what's more, I met him when I weighed 195 pounds and he liked me, he really liked me. It was finally time for the princess to get her prince. Read on my friends.

Chapter 8
My Godsend, Jeff

I know at this point of my story I could continue to talk about my battles with weight and self-esteem. I could – but I won't – at least for now. It's time to interject a little fairy tale princess into my story because what happened at this stage of life was like a dream come true.

Some people may have been told that, from birth, God had made a person for them to marry and love unconditionally. God had a plan for people to live "happily ever after." As young child I truly believed that God was holding on to someone for me. Maybe part of me believed that I did not lose the weight before because "it" was really going to happen; or that I was challenging the "idea" to see if someone would really love me as I was. I'm not really sure which it was.

When I was very young, maybe three years of age, I was shopping with Mom and Grandma in a department store. I was a girly girl and loved ruffled, lacey, and frilly clothes. I remember telling Mom that she should buy some frilly clothes and Grandma laughed. Mom dressed conservatively and classically and was not into trendy, frilly things. Grandma told me, "One day when you find your true love, I will buy those frilly clothes for you." It was like a fairy tale for me and I spent thousands of hours dreaming of that day, even as a young child.

I wanted the fairy tale as a young child and into my adulthood, too. I wished and prayed for it to come true. Truthfully, until I was 28, I never even had that feeling. In both of my serious relationships up to that point, I never heard the "heavenly romantic music" I had always imagined or felt that "feeling." I thought I loved both men in my past and that they were the ones that screwed up and lost me. Honestly I never knew what true love really was except that of motherly love for Torri and family love for my parents, brothers, and other close relatives.

At points in my life, I just gave up on the heavenly romantic music

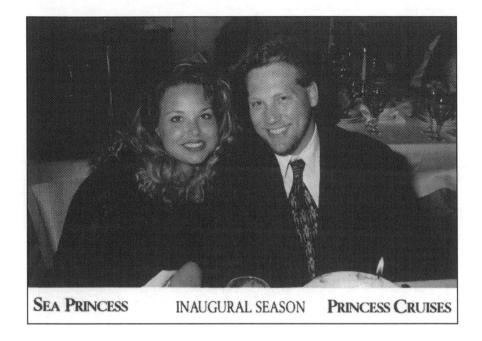

SEA PRINCESS　　　INAUGURAL SEASON　　PRINCESS CRUISES

or the feeling of truly being in love with a wonderful man. I had always settled for less because I wanted to be loved and cared for. Was there really any such thing as heavenly music and true love? Or was all of this stuff that only happened in fairy tales? All of us know that fairy tales never come true; they are just make believe to entertain our children.

Well, I was wrong! God does make one person for us and I finally found him. There is heavenly music and there is true love. I finally got that feeling. But it took a quick reality check to convince me. At first I thought I was having a premature hot flash as I had many, many female issues. But after checking it out with my doctor, she convinced me I was not beginning menopause at 28. I was smitten.

I met Jeffrey James Wengle, my future Prince Charming, at a party that my friend invited me to around the New Year. This was at the time I had recently moved in with my brother and had separated from Tom. I first arrived at the party and checked my coat. I felt a cold draft come in behind me and turned to look at who was coming in. It was my girlfriend who had brought a male friend. I barely looked at or spoke to my friend; rather, I looked right into the eyes of her friend, Jeffrey James. Our eyes met in unison, just like in a movie (no kidding). It was in slow motion too! I can't explain it – it's just the way it happened.

I was wearing a shorter, slightly flowered skirt with a sweater twin set, black heels, and my most prized possession: a long camel coat with a fur collar. I still have that coat in my closet. It is a size 18 but I can't bear to part with it. It is a souvenir from that magical night. I always think I am going to get it altered and wear it again. But I am definitely not giving it up.

The three of us sat together and began to talk. I felt so weird, not knowing how to behave, like a little girl. I wound up trying to blow Jeff off. I didn't know how to analyze my feelings except to rationalize them as indigestion from the pizza I ate at lunch. No matter, Jeff wouldn't stop staring at me.

I moved down a few chairs to talk with some other folks yet there was Jeff, still staring at me from the end of the table. The big moment in my life had arrived and I was blowing it – because I was blown away by it. I had to leave the table because I felt strange and my heart raced. Maybe I took too many diet pills that day, I just couldn't remember. That had to be some rationalization for this, right?

I went into the ladies room. My face was flushed and I was sweating. What the heck, maybe I had the flu. I definitely was not sure what was going on, I just hoped it wasn't anything serious. Maybe it was a bug. More appropriately, a love bug.

I grabbed a drink and talked with my girlfriend. I needed all the dirt I could gather on Jeff. She said he was going through a divorce and that she really liked him. Uh oh. She knew him through her job and he lived in Brighton, the city I wanted to live in. A scary coincidence?

We were standing near the dance floor, talking and taking in the party atmosphere. As I turned around to look at the dance floor, Jeff was right behind me. He wanted to dance. No way!

Because I was overweight growing up, I really never danced much. I took tap lessons in second grade. For some reason, the tap number, "We come from Mars," didn't prepare me for dancing that night.

The DJ was playing some fast dance music and I was somewhat mortified. I was trying to find an excuse – any excuse – for not dancing but Jeff wouldn't take no for an answer. He said, "Don't worry. Every song is a slow song." I liked his logic. So we danced slowly to a fast song. People were bumping into us; maybe they didn't like our slow pace. And the music was too loud to carry on a conversation. The DJ finally slowed it down and we danced some more – this time with the ability to hear each other talk.

I'm glad we did. Jeff gave me the "scoop" on him and my girlfriend. Jeff said he told her he would prefer to be friends. He was in the middle

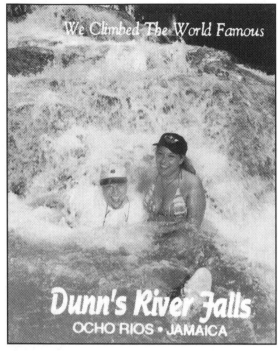

We Climbed The World Famous

Dunn's River Falls
OCHO RIOS • JAMAICA

of a divorce and wasn't interested in a new relationship. Whew – just friends. That was good to know since I really didn't want a serious relationship either. Ha.

I was still pretty nervous about the evening and not sure how to handle my emotions. The two combined made me opt for an early exit from the party. I wanted to get out of this "situation" fast. I was a runner when I felt uncomfortable – not in the physical, put on a pair of running shoes sense – I just want to get out in a hurry.

I felt like slipping out unnoticed but Jeff chased me into the coatroom. He gave me his business card and asked if I would call him the next week. I said yes. He kissed me goodnight. The kiss was not a peck on the cheek. It was a good kiss on the lips. I felt a little dizzy and nauseous after the smooch, not knowing if I really was getting sick or really was falling in love. If I was really sick, I hoped that Jeff wouldn't catch it. If I was really sick in love, well, that is a different story. It would be okay for Jeff to catch that illness.

I didn't call him the next week but he tracked me down anyway. Maybe I wanted to play a little hard-to-get. That guy was scaring me. I didn't know what was wrong, but I felt sick around Jeff – or I thought it was a sickness. But part of me was happy he called, because I would have never called him. We talked for a couple hours and whined to each other about our soon-to-be ex-spouses. We also learned a ton about each other. He wanted to meet up but I was swamped with work and Torri. I had no time to really begin a relationship – or so I thought. Torri needed me too and I could not imagine starting another relationship when I was just getting out of my marriage. Jeff was a gentleman, knowing that seeing each other while we were each still legally married might not look good. We were both concerned how our families and friends would react.

Our feelings of propriety did not stop us from talking on the phone – daily. We learned a lot during these conversations. The one thing I obsessed about was our physical makeup. Jeff was almost six foot tall and weighed 183. I weighed 195 on a short frame. I thought to myself, "Surely I could not date anyone that weighed less than me." That was a big deal to me and I could not do it.

So, I did what any sensible person would do. I began dieting hot and heavy again. I had taken a month off of really trying to lose weight over the holidays and was not taking my full strength of diet pills. But I didn't gain any weight during this time. Of course, I didn't lose any either.

I liked Jeff a lot. I knew there was something there. Part of me was scared. I'd have crazy thoughts of how Jeff was plotting to use me and then leave me, which made me pull away from him. I wouldn't answer his calls and he would be forced to chase me down. It was not fair to him, but I honestly did not know what I was doing. I had never been pursued like this before and felt uneasy.

It took me two-three months of dieting to get down to Jeff's weight: 183. When that happened I decided it was time to "celebrate" and set up a dinner date with Jeff. We met for dinner at Chili's in Brighton in early March.

I missed him and he missed me. We had not seen each other in a while, but it was like we never missed a beat. Our eyes met and we did not stop staring at each other for two hours (except the few times I caught him staring down my suit coat). I was dressed to the nine's, had my hair done, make-up just right, and wore high heels. I felt pretty good about myself. My "normal skinny" was 183 and all was good.

We had a wonderful time. The music from the restaurant played in my head and the special "feeling" was definitely there. At that point I knew I was not physically sick – it was love sickness.

Jeff walked me to my truck. We kissed and sure enough, that dizziness came back. He grabbed me to make sure I wouldn't fall over. I guess he recognized the return of my hot flashes. Or did I have some physical ailment like an inner ear infection? Nope.

I kept thinking about him, this guy named Jeffrey James. He had blond hair and bluish eyes. He was two years older than me yet he retained his boyish looks. In fact knowing what I know now about him now, his face had that seventh grade look, the year he began to part his hair on the side.

Jeff was clean cut with short hair, classic dresser with good shoes, educated from a well known engineering school, and began his own business, a company called Adtran, with a childhood friend after graduating from college.

This all sounds wonderful and almost too good to be true. So naturally I spent many sleepless nights trying to figure out what was wrong with him. Obviously something had to be wrong. I just couldn't figure out if he was genuine or if he was playing me.

I was so scared at times. I hate to admit it, but I ran a couple times. Actually I ran for the first several years of our relationship (not physically running, mentally running), but Jeff kept reassuring me and kept chasing me.

I asked Jeff the two 'W's" – why and when he fell in love with me. He said he fell in love with me the first time our eyes met. He said it was like each of us saw into each other souls. He said I was larger than life and he wasn't talking about my size. He thought I was confident and beautiful.

Look out world! The music started playing again and I began flashing again. Now this is what I called LOVE. I was convinced. Now it was time to do some planning. I had separated from Tom in September and moved most of my stuff out by Christmas. I know this probably wasn't the best idea, but Jeff took my dog Calie (her real name Victoria's Caliginous Gem) with him for a few months, until Torri and I got on our feet. It just so happened that we were both looking for houses and decided to get one together instead. I know it seemed like a whirlwind – and it was. We made plans for Torri and I to move to Howell (one town from Brighton) in the summer and purchased a house together.

Looking back now, it seemed like a rash decision, mainly because of Torri. She was seven years old and a little apprehensive. I told her that I understood how she felt and I that I would never let anyone or anything come between us. Torri was number one. If she didn't like the new home; we would move. But I could see she was getting excited about meeting Jeff and seeing Calie again. I showed her pictures of her new house and pictures of Calie. I also told her that Jeff's dog, Nick would be part of the household.

Torri tells me now that she was scared, but excited. She and I had moved a lot. Tom was still fresh in her mind and she was unsure of all men – not trusting them and fearing they might not treat her Mom well. But my promise of moving again if she was uncomfortable made her feel less anxious.

The big moving day had arrived. Torri and I had my truck loaded and we headed to Howell. Howell is a rural community, about 45 miles west of Detroit. It had lots of land and trees, not anything like the city living I was used to and 50' wide lots we had lived on. As we were driving through our cute little new town, Torri saw this huge mansion and grounds. Howell people called it the McPherson Mansion. The big white historic home had tennis courts and barns. Torri said, "Mom, maybe we could live there if I don't like Jeff." I appeased her and said, "Okay, let's see how it goes first."

We pulled up into the driveway of our own pretty big house, which included five acres for Torri to play and run with the dogs. Calie was so happy to see Torri that she knocked down Torri and licked her face for what seemed like 5 minutes. Nick was curious, too. He had just gotten used to living with Calie and along comes a seven-year-old kid. It was understandable that he was a little standoffish at first.

Eventually, Torri and the dogs began playing and running around the huge yard while Jeff helped me unload the truck. Jeff and Torri met for the first time. Torri, who was shy at the time, was gripping my arm – tight. Jeff came down to her level and they shook hands. Jeff showed Torri where Nick and Calie's softballs and Frisbee's were – in the garage. And Jeff handed Torri one, to see if both dogs run for one toy. Calie was much faster, but Nick had more determination. It was cute. Torri loved Nick. He was such a handsome "boy" and he was really big. Jeff took Torri in the house to see her room; I hung out in the garage, unpacking a little. Shortly after, Torri ran out, saying how big her room was and that Jeff was going to build her some seats for her dormer windows – and maybe a bookcase.

Torri and Jeff hit it off. They were both cautious a little at first, but it did not take long at all for Torri to play and trust Jeff.

During the first day I went outside to check on Torri. She was sitting on the grass talking to Calie. Torri said, "Calie, I think we are going to like this house and Jeff. But if we don't, Mommy is going to buy us a mansion." I laughed and hugged her. Torri was such a sweetie, to other people and kids. And she loved animals. She would sit and talk to her animals and hold their heads up so she could see their eyes. Even as a baby she held up Muffin's face, our first dog, so she could look right into the eyes.

I had a room upstairs, next to Torri's. Jeff slept in the master bedroom on the first floor. There were a couple of reasons for this. Torri was only seven. She had always been in the room next to mine. And I was a paranoid Mom. What if there was a fire and the stairway was blocked? I wasn't sure if Torri could open the window, drop the fire ladder, and make it out. We also have a bonus room on the second floor which is our family room. Jeff and I would spend time up there while Torri was falling asleep. Being upstairs with her made her feel more comfortable and she settled in nicely. Torri loved her huge room. It also had an attached room that we used for all her toys.

I was a good Mom, but always doing too much for Torri. Jeff saw it and we had to make adjustments. Torri couldn't even make toast at age seven – because of her overprotective mom. Jeff taught Torri how to cook, clean, and help out around the house. I sheltered Torri out of guilt.

The first year was really magical for all of us. Torri and I still talk about that first meeting and the beginning of our adventure and new life. She always said it was the right decision and that she trusted me despite all of the crap we had both been through together.

Jeff is who Torri calls Dad; and who will most likely walk her down the aisle on her wedding day, at least as of this writing she says so. They have so much in common and honestly, I think sometimes, she likes Jeff more than me.

Jeff is even tempered, explaining to Torri for seemingly hours on end any family problems or concerns. He is a good listener and gives Torri options rather than yelling at her or telling her what to do, like one former housemate who shall remain nameless. Tom. They giggle and laugh all the time.

Even through the terrible teenage years, Jeff has been our rock. Sometimes I wonder if I could have ever done it without him. He helped me when Torri was sick with flus, stayed home with her if she had to miss school, drove her to her events or after school activities, helped her with her homework, especially math, and loved her when she needed a man's love. Torri wasn't the only one who felt loved. I still heard the music in my head and felt that "feeling."

Yes, I doubted whether God's "plan" for me was real or not. And if I ever questioned God's plan, I am truly sorry. God has been protecting me and watching me my whole life, fully knowing his whole plan for me. At times I doubted the plan – but not any more. I still wonder what's next in his plan, but I don't doubt him.

I believe God made Jeff for me and Torri. Torri needed a strong male role model, to see how marriage and partnerships really work. He shows how much a man can love his daughter, even if it is not a biological tie (although everyone thinks Torri looks like Jeff and people think Jeff and

I look like brother and sister). We have a wonderful family life now – not perfect of course – but wonderful and we all know we are unconditionally loved.

Our life together was just beginning and our future was bright. Jeff was going to have a family and a woman that was more like an equal partner than a mate. I was going to have a man that just loved me, as I was. And Torri was going to see how a father really loves his daughter.

Chapter 9
A Great Threesome

The union of Jeff, Torri, and I in 1999 started a whole new, exciting chapter in my life. It was a magical time filled with new feelings and new memories. I barely remember my life without Jeff. All of the bad times were shoved to the background. Even now I think about many events that Jeff was seemingly a part of but he gently reminds me, "No honey, that was not me." And then I realize it was with Mike or Tom. I was acting like a graphic artist, superimposing Jeff's face on the bodies of long forgotten men. The memories are much better with Jeff in them.

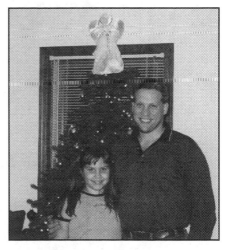

Jeff and I really felt no need to ever marry, but our families wanted us to be "legal'" – in the real and in the spiritual sense. And it was the thing to do for Torri, too. With that said, Jeff put a big rock on my hand in 2000 to show others that I was "taken." There were no wedding plans at the time but the big event would be inevitable. I had some very important issues to iron out at this point in my life, namely, would we add any more kids to our union. I believe everyone should have the option of having kids, and I did imagine a little Jeffy walking around the house. Although I was content with just having Torri, I couldn't be the one to decide to never give Jeff his own baby. Jeff confided that he never wanted children of his own, even though I gave him one last chance to change his mind. I said I would have a baby with him – but he had to act quickly. I wanted to be a young energetic

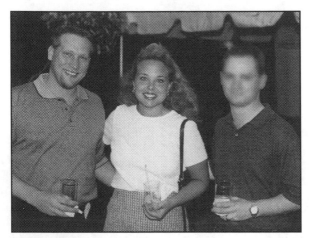 Mom and I was afraid of how the weight gain would affect me physically and emotionally.

I did have concerns about Torri feeling left out. Having a baby is magical and it would have been possible for some of that magic to overwhelm Torri. Jeff and I didn't want that. He adored Torri and didn't want their closeness to be jeopardized. Jeff decided he was happy with our family the way it was – and I was happy to concur. And even though Torri would have loved to have a little brother or sister, she was okay with our decision.

With that said, I can safely summarize how our last ten years have been – wonderful. True, we have had our struggles but a lot of love and caring can help to overcome anything. If anything, I was the one who brought the excess baggage – literally – to the relationship. But even though I had struggled with weight issues for so long, including well into our marriage, the problems didn't seem so bad, because Jeff loved me for me – and he had been a real trooper adding me and Torri to his life.

In the first stages of our relationship I struggled with my weight. Although I had never looked better, I wanted to weigh less. I was down to 175 by the time we moved to Howell, but I was the heaviest girl Jeff had ever dated. His ex-wife was tall and thin and I was not. I struggled with that internally. Actually, I struggled with everything internally, not letting Jeff into some of my thoughts. I had grown up not letting people know how I was really feeling. I put on a good front, always seemed chipper and bubbly, but I was struggling inside.

For the first few years of our relationship I truly believed that Jeff would leave me some day. I really felt that happiness – for me – was only fleeting and that this relationship would end up like the others. Jeff had never even hinted at it or behaved like it would happen. I just assumed it would.

I should have been tipped off all along about Jeff's compassion and care for me. He loved to touch me! Jeff is a touchy, feely hugger. I really hadn't been hugged and cuddled by anyone like that. He laughs today, but he often talks about how bad I used to hug him. Luckily for him – and me – I am now an excellent hugger. Jeff taught me how to hug and be affectionate. I believe this show of affection has also made me a better wife, mother, daughter, sister, aunt, and friend. My own family is closer and "huggier" – or at least it seemed since I "converted." We all say we love each other over the phone and write gushy notes in birthday cards and holiday cards. It is wonderful now. Maybe it always was wonderful but it took Jeff's love to help me recognize it.

In bed, he always wanted to spoon, laying on the side, facing the same direction and holding on, or just be touching me while we slept. Jeff would be snoring away and there I was, wide-eyed in panic mode. The constant touching was difficult and very strange for me. I would stay up all most all night having panic attacks.

Not only was touchy-feely foreign to me, so was good communication. I would be mad at something and hold it in, unable to express my anger or to vent. Or if I was mad, I wanted to be left alone. These characteristics are totally opposite of Jeff's. He would follow me around trying to get inside my head. Jeff wanted to help me, but I didn't know how to communicate on his level. I could not even explain to him what I was feeling. I knew I felt anxious or in a panic mode, but could not articulate what was wrong.

Realistically, many of my "problems" came down to my weight and body image. I felt I did not deserve a normal, educated guy, or felt he would eventually leave me because of my body. This went on for years.

Also, when we began to live together I weighed 175 and within a year I lost another 40 pounds, where I remain today. Funny thing (and frustrating) – it did not matter, I still felt fat. I still had issues with my body and I still drove Jeff nuts with my lack of communication and closeness that a wife should share with her husband. Poor Jeff, he wasn't the problem; I was. Or to be more exact, my body was.

Besides being a little messed up in the head, I was messed up in the stomach too. I was starving – hungry all of the time. Once Metabolife was banned due to the Ephedrine, I had nothing to keep my hunger pains in check. So I was hungry and crabby. If there were ever reasons for Jeff to walk out on me, he had plenty. I was not fun to be around.

While I was dieting I was eating 300-500 calories a day, which made me miserable. Even when I ate healthy foods and added a few more calories, I would gain weight. My metabolism was shot. I would fluctuate from 135-142 pounds, sometimes as high as 145. My mood for the day depend-

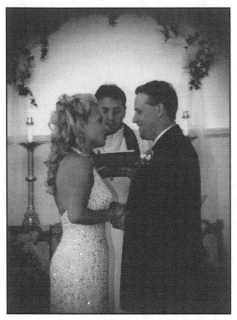

ed on what I weighed that morning before work. If it was high, I was miserable. If it was low, I was happier but hungry. This went on for years.

Around 2001, Jeff kept talking with me about working out – and how it would help my overall disposition. So, in 2002 I took up Tai Kwon Do with Torri. It made me feel better but it just wasn't for me. The experiment only lasted a couple of months. Plus I really didn't think I had the time to devote to working out. After all, I worked full-time, driving 1-1/2 or two hours each way to work. I often would have to return to my job in the evenings and do more – the role of a manager never stopped. I was also mentoring other people, too. On top of work, I was responsible for seeing that Torri was always where she had to be – and that I was a good Mom.

There were other things more important to do than working out, especially after Jeff and I bought a commercial building in August 2001. We

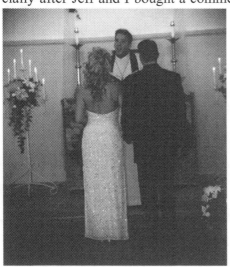

eventually opened our Livingston Antique Outlet in June 2002. We worked tirelessly on our 20,000 (now 33,000) square foot building, doing all the work ourselves. Once the mall opened I quit Nextel and Jeff sold his company. Jeff labored and I ran the business side of the mall.

Somewhere in the middle of all of this – May 10th, 2002 – we managed to finally get married. We were married in a historical chapel in our small town of Howell. We had 52 of our family and friends celebrate the event with us. We were back at home by 9:00 p.m., because we had to work at our store the next morning. How romantic. But it was a very special, un-stressful, relaxing day, the way a wedding day should be and usually isn't. We didn't doubt our decision, especially since we had been living the same lifestyle of a married couple. Our families supported us fully. In fact, our friends wondered why we took so long to tie the knot. I look back at those pictures with huge grins, and have oodles of those pictures of our wedding day all over the house. Even our two dogs, Calie and Nick are featured in our wedding album and their pictures from that day are throughout our house, even though they have both passed away. I made the right decision – and Jeff was legally bound to me. Try leaving me now!

Later that year, around Christmas, things got a little tense. To be blunt, Jeff had it out with me. No, he didn't leave me but the threat was there. Why? Because of everything I had complained about before: my weight and my hunger. He said, "Listen, you are crabby and miserable because you don't eat enough food. I don't care how much you weigh, but you need to eat more food Lori! Torri and I (they teamed up on me) are going to leave you unless you change."

Huh? My husband and daughter are going to leave me if I don't eat more food? That sounds like something I could write a book about. Ahem.

Although the truth hurts, I knew they were right and I had to make changes. Jeff and Torri are my life, and I am not going to lose them, ever.

In an effort to speed up these changes, Jeff showed me pictures of his first girlfriend. She looked a lot like me when I was chubby – and she was short like me too. Jeff explained if I would have stayed the same weight from when we met, he would still be with me today. Why? Because he loves who I am: Lori. He loved me, not what I looked like, but me. He loved my work ethic, my partnership in business, my love of animals, my love for our families, and our love for each other.

He told me I was his soul mate and he could not live without me. He couldn't even remember what life was like (much quieter, I am sure) without me. He genuinely did not care what I weighed. I don't think that sunk in for a while. I remember walking around the house, thinking, "Jeff really doesn't care what I weigh." This is what I hoped for as a child and teen, to be married to a man that loved me for me and did not care what I weighed. Even at this point in my life and in the very back of my head, I thought Jeff would leave me if I gained the weight back. What a huge mental relief that day brought me.

Jeff talked to me about working out. I said I would look into some gyms and hinted that a membership might make a nice gift. For Christmas, Jeff bought Torri and me a membership at the Howell Fitness Center. Jeff went in and met the owner, Dale Sr., and received a tour. It was a family run business, non-intimidating, and his dogs came to work with him. Now this was a person I could identify with!

That present of the gym membership once again changed my world for the better.

Chapter 10
Beginning to Change My World

The next paths I chose to follow involved two very different ways to tone up and shape up. The first, weight training is one that I recommend as the preferred way to get in shape. At the time I really began weight training I believed that working hard, I could look like a swimsuit model, even after years of abuse and weight gains and loss. Because I was relatively young, I really didn't think I would be left with extra skin hanging from my body. I was in my early 30s and surely my body would bounce back (actually bounce forward as I was never at a healthy weight). But years of yo-yo dieting, starving, and gaining the weight back took its toll on my body, especially my skin. So the second path I ended up with, after four years of working out consistently, ended up to be surgery. But this path – for anyone – should only be used as a last resort measure. I'll explain both.

Weight training became the real answer for me, something that many other people already knew. I realized I was able to change my shape quickly. What I didn't realize is that it would become a "good" addiction. The more results I saw, the harder I worked. I am not afraid to work hard, but this, well, this was so addicting.

I began by taking a jumpstart class that was planned by a personal trainer. I really learned some good things. This class was put on by a trainer that had experience in training people to work out with weights. She began by testing us to see where our fitness level was that day. It was fun. I flunked many of the fitness tests, such as pushup, reach test, and so on. I was very unhealthy. This jumpstart was designed to get a person started quickly. There was no time to be babied. But we also learned a lot about our bodies. Unfortunately, our trainer moved to Arizona during the class and we were all left hanging – skin and all.

At least I now had a better understanding of my health situation. I was feeling better with more energy. As a bonus, I was less tired and crabby. My only problem was because I had only learned a few routines. I ended up doing the same exercises, weight lifting, and sets and reps every time I went to the gym. And the results began very positively. I was becoming strong, during the first six weeks of exercise, then, my progress began to slow down and almost no new improvement was realized. I continued these same exercises for about ten months doing the same repetitions until I realized I needed another fitness trainer to replace my original one.

That October (2003) I hired a new personal trainer and in six weeks of twice-a-week workouts, I saw fantastic results. I saw similar results in six weeks versus those I had achieved in ten months. I was thinking this was truly a miracle.

But there was still a problem. My trainer did not want to teach me how to train myself. I became dependent on her for my fitness. I'll admit that I was partly to blame but it seemed that some of the training should have been geared to "one-on-none" interaction, if you know what I mean. I ended up getting hurt a few times, but continued on with her for a couple years. I would go for a few visits and then work on my own – and keep repeating the cycle.

I also began buying a lot of fitness books and magazines. Reading is such a great training method in itself. I learned how to control my own destiny from the words on each page. I began to understand why trainers saw results and learned about muscle confusion. Not letting your muscles get used to one routine is so important, which is why trainers don't do the same routine week after week. In fact, my trainer trained me on so many exercises I could barely remember how to perform them with out her. So I rationalized my need for constant monitoring – geesh.

However, as time went on, I began to figure out how to achieve great results in weight training on my own. I became my own guinea pig. I found books with exercises and learned why/how to use them effectively. I needed to gain knowledge on all aspects of weight training in order to perform correctly. Learning about form and accuracy, speed, weight and reps became much clearer. I had finally found the solution!

I would go to the gym on a regular basis three-four days a week. In the beginning Torri was with me all the time. She even followed my lead, too. We both had our doubts and weren't sure the workouts were really working. But eventually we realized we were doing it correctly, as lifting weights has a way of catching up to you days later. Also, because we did a lot of new exercises, we received the value of muscle confusion. Our bodies were not used to working out those muscles in that particular way. It's like when you go outside and weed your flower bed. The next day you can barely tie your shoes. Muscle confusion is an awesome tool; it keeps your body guessing.

Where was Jeff during all of this? He was usually rubbing my sore body nightly, working out all the knots I had created. Not only did Jeff ensure I could leave our mall early for the workouts, he would also cook, clean, and do laundry. He saw my results, not just physically, but how I was feeling mentally and would do anything to ensure Torri and I made it to the gym at least three times a week. Sometimes we fell off the wagon and Jeff would pick us back up and shove us out the door – not because he felt we needed it for weight loss but because after our workout, we felt like a million dollars. He wanted us to be happy. Jeff's motto, Happy Wife, Happy Life. Corny, but effective.

I really didn't do much cardio during this period I enjoyed challenging my muscles with weight training. Cardio is aerobic exercise which involves or improves oxygen consumption by the body. Aerobic means "with oxygen," and refers to the use of oxygen in the body's metabolic or energy-generating process. Many types of exercise are aerobic, and by definition are performed at moderate levels of intensity for extended periods of time. That is the technical term. I say cardio is weight training for your heart and lungs. Hey, if we want to live, we need a healthy heart and respiratory system. At the time I found cardio monotonous and boring – I couldn't get motivated. I performed by weight training in a 'circuit training' atmosphere which is short for "no rest." I liked that better but now I am a bonafide cardio nut.

Some days I overdid my weight training. I wouldn't be able to walk down the stairs in the morning. When I tried to get out of bed, my abs hurt so bad that I had to roll to the side instead of lifting up in the air.

Although I did not lose any more weight, everyone "thought" I was still losing. Why? Because muscle weighs more than fat and if you add lean muscle, you will condense your body into a streamline machine. I did lose a size or two, but no weight on the scale. I could wear styles of clothes I never thought I would be able to wear. Overall, it was great. My confidence grew and I was pretty comfortable with myself – finally!

The theory behind weight training working is this: While resting, you burn one calorie per one pound of fat; you burn 35 calories per one pound of muscle while resting. So if you took five pounds of fat and turned it into five pounds of muscle, you would burn an extra 175 calories per day. That equates to over 45,000 calories a year, which equates to 18.2 pounds lost in a year. You can do all of this without changing your eating habits.

Weight training was the answer I had been looking for my whole life. It was – and is – fun and not boring. It is invigorating and has helped lower my blood pressure, change my shape, gave me confidence in my body and myself – and I felt great!

Ah, but as the late and great radio broadcaster Paul Harvey would say, "And now, the rest of the story." It is time to talk about the second way I "toned up" and not the recommended one – surgery.

At this point in my life I had a few issues left. I had very nice abs. From about two inches below my belly button all the way up to my rib cage, I looked great. I was getting lines in my abs and I could wear a half top, which I did, often. But two inches below my waist and below my privates, I had a flap of very thin, disgusting, stretch marked, nasty skin that flapped over my pubic area. In clothes it appeared I had an almost flat stomach, but out of clothes I had hanging old bag of skin.

I also had a noticeable problem with my inner and outer thighs. I had three folds of skin down my inner thigh. The first one, was about a three-inch fold, the second was 1-1/2 inches and the third maybe a half-inch. My outer thigh had a blob of fat I referred to as my "saddle bag." Giddy- up. It was only a three-to-four inch diameter, but no matter what I did, it would not go away. I later learned that it was part of my butt that moved to the side, and I learned how to improve that look later on.

Other trainers told me I could keep working on it, which I did for an-other year. But it was frustrating and fruitless. Finally, I went to a plastic surgeon and he told me that I was down to skin and bones. Yes me, stand-ing there naked in front of a plastic surgeon and smiling because he said I was skin and bones! He said that no matter what, I could not get rid of extra skin. I had always carried my weight in my hips, thighs and lower abs – and my butt. And now I was paying the price, no pun intended as you will see in a moment.

Jeff was not happy to hear his prognosis. We expected a tummy tuck but not an inner thigh lift. An inner thigh lift is a cut in the crease of your inner thigh about fifteen inches long from front to back on both sides. I explained to Jeff that my folds of skin would never go away, unless I was to gain a lot of weight back, which was not an option for me. Also, this inner thigh lift would help my outer thigh saddlebag enough and if I continued to work out I would be happy with the results. My outer thigh problems bothered me a lot, but I was not afraid to work them out through cardio and weight training. Remember, I said I was addicted to weight training and its results – I wanted to continue to improve my overall look and psyche.

Now the kicker: the surgery would cost $16,000 and was not covered by our medical insurance. On top of that, I was not guaranteed to lose any size or weight. Because my problems were skin, very thin skin, I would remain the same weight and size. I had to get over that; there was nothing wrong with my size, just how I felt naked, or in swimsuits. But there were 16,000 reasons why I shouldn't have done this, too.

With Jeff's support, I went ahead with the surgery in 2006. The procedure took a whopping six hours. Jeff was such a trooper. He stayed with me before the surgery and watched as I began shaking prior to going into the operating room. Jeff held my hand and reassured me. Even at the last moment I was having second thoughts about the inner thigh lift. I was scared Jeff told me he would always love me no matter what. Maybe it was the "no matter what" part that had me scared the most.

After the surgery, I woke up to him holding my hand again. He kissed me and said the doctor told him it went very well. My nurse taught me how to push a button for morphine pain medicine to go into my IV. I never pushed the button. Why? I don't know, maybe it was because I was overcome with joy. Even swollen and wrapped I could tell that my saddle bags looked better and my stomach was tighter and flatter all the way down. I was elated! Having skin removed for any reason, especially those involving weight loss, is a big deal. In my case, it helped me feel whole and normal – something I hadn't felt for most of my life.

Jeff took me home the next morning and did everything for me, I mean everything. My inner thigh incisions were a little tough and we had to clean them and re-tape them. I had drainage tubes in my lower abdomen that Jeff had to empty every so often for 10 days. I could barely move and using the bathroom was a real chore. You can only imagine the things my man did for me. Jeff brought me a wooden chair from our pole building so I could sit and take a shower, he shaved my legs as I could not bend that far down, and he washed my hair as it hurt to move around a lot. He did anything and everything I needed – talk about the "for better or worse" vow. Jeff also took care of our four animals, woke up early to drive Torri to school and pick her up, made us all our meals, and cleaned the house. What a man!

Jeff stayed with me for a week until I was ready to be home by myself. I never saw Jeff so happy to go back to work – go figure. He said I was a trooper, which I was. I figured since I was the one who wanted it, I was not entitled to whine about it. Of course, the pain medicine they gave me was great. I was mostly out of it the first three-four days and slept a lot.

Now, to my point. Women ask me all the time if plastic surgery is the answer. I tell them it is a personal issue. For me, because I gained and lost and gained and lost and did that so many times, I really had no other choice. The areas I had carried the majority of my weight, upper arms (on my list maybe one day), lower abs and thighs, were never going to look as I wanted them to look. That extra skin made me still feel fat or out of shape and I could not stop obsessing about it. I worked out so hard, for so long and I needed this to make me happy. I was prepared emotionally – and financially – for the surgery.

If you are thinking about surgery, go see a board certified plastic surgeon. My surgeon specialized in Bariatrics, which are surgical procedures to band off or remove part of the stomach and redirect some of the intestines. Patients who have had this procedure can lose over 100 pounds. Many of those people have been very obese for long periods of time and this surgery is their last resort. I have had several clients that have done this and it is major surgery. If I did not lose the weight and it was readily available, I would have done this, too. Some of my doctor's patients had lost 80-200 pounds. I would also advise you to do your homework through research. Look at some of their clients before and after, ask lots of questions. If you choose surgery, follow the pre- and post-surgery rules to the letter. If your areas are not that bad and can be changed through exercise, think twice about the surgery. It's expensive and dangerous. You end up with a scar and the recovery takes four-six weeks.

My inner thigh lift is usually performed on people with severe issues – usually people that lost more weight than I did. But my doctor said I was an unusual case and he had never seen anything like mine. There was my justification – I was an original.

My inner thigh scar is almost gone after three years. It looks better compared to how it looked before surgery and now is a thin line almost invisible, unless you get right next to it. It appears as a light pencil mark almost. My tummy tuck scar is still there a little bit more than my inner thigh lift, but it's in an area no one is supposed to see anyway. And most importantly, I am happy with the results.

I have had clients that have had tummy tucks. My advice to everyone is to lose all of the weight first and then have the surgery. Understand, you will not have flat abs from surgery alone, you will have to work out to attain really firm, flat abs. Tummy tucks are designed to tighten skin, remove extra skin, remove stretch marks, and flatten the belly in general. But you have to keep working out or your efforts may all be for naught.

So, I was hooked on weight lifting and had my surgery. And one more thing, I used my recovery time, lying on the couch to take an online class to become a personal trainer. What a great way to utilize my downtime and further my dreams. Anything and everything I had ever wanted was coming true. As a kid, I use to dream of losing all my weight and then teaching people my secrets just like Richard Simmons. Well now I was going to inspire all kinds of people. And once they saw my results, they would know they could do it, too.

Before I continue with my story, I want to a moment to interject an interesting event that convinced me I had made the right decision to lose weight and tone up. So let's fast forward to 2008.

In 2008 I went to my 20 year high school reunion. No one knew who I was. Former classmates thought it was Jeff who went to my school. Once the word got out, the whispering and pointing began. My old classmates came up to me – to see if it was really me. They only recognized my voice, my eyes, and my "tan." Some of the formerly popular girls had gotten fat or just were not happy with their lives. They were the ones who didn't bother to say hello. My core group of friends from high school was still fabulous and funny. My friends said that now I was officially the "hottest" girl from our class. Physical change is one thing, internal growth is another. I was lucky to be among friends who believed in both.

My class was proud of me. And here is the best part. Kevin my former crush since 9th grade, was talking in a group about 20 feet from me. I heard, "no way" really loud. A group of men had heard who I was. One of them was Kevin, the boy that used to threaten to pick me up and throw me in the garbage, in a nice way. He was always nice to me, and I thought he even liked me back then. Kevin walked over to me and said, "Lori Ellul (maiden name), you are beautiful, but you were always beautiful." How about that to top off my already wonderful night? I wanted to hear those words so badly at my reunion, even envisioning it twenty years earlier. I dreamt of losing all my weight and coming back to comments and whispers – just like it happened. Jeff always tells me to be careful what I wish for. But on this night my wish came true and nothing else mattered.

You too, can have this moment in your life. It might not be at a high school reunion, but something similar. Working out with weights correctly, using cardio, and adhering to a program will make all your dreams come true – and you will feel good doing it.

Now, let's turn back to "the rest of the story."

Chapter 11
Becoming a Personal Trainer

My online course to become a personal trainer was a nice diversion to my recovery from surgery. Over the next year I studied each chapter and learned the coursework, often researching items on my own. And every night I would go try out on myself what I learned. The coursework was not hard. It made sense to me and I breezed right through the chapters. Once I took each test, I was sent more books to read. And so on.

I was obsessed with everything regarding fitness, from new exercise equipment to fitness infomercials and products. I bought and read everything I could during that year. Once I received my certificate, I wanted more. It wasn't enough that I had just one certification. I wanted a special certification from a really good personal training organization.

I researched each of the certificates I had thought about getting and decided on The American Council on Exercise, who are recognized as the watchdogs on exercise for Americans. The book and study material was overwhelming and frankly, I didn't know if I could absorb and remember all of the material.

I studied almost 40-50 hours a week for over two months and finally passed my test. I was now an ACE Certified Personal Trainer and so proud of it. I mean really, really proud of it. My life had done a 360 degree turn during the "Jeff time period" and I was more determined than ever to keep moving onward and upward.

I began to advertise my new business, "Get Your Skinny, Personal Training," showing my before and after shots, and boy did I fill up my schedule. I primarily thought I would only train women, but no, the men came and so did the teens.

My philosophy was very clear to my clients: add muscle, raise your metabolism, and burn fat, baby! I instilled everything I had learned into my clients. I made my clients get off their couches and move every day. I taught my clients why, so they remembered to do it on their own, a lesson I had learned on my own.

I loved being a personal trainer. I had always wanted a job to help others. One of my original goals in college was to become a child psychologist and help kids through tough times. I had wanted to be a child psychologist based on my experience after my parents were divorced. They sent me to see Dr. Doyle, a child psychologist. He played games with me every week and I thought to myself, "Gee, it must be nice to be paid to play Monopoly with kids." Also, at the end of our sessions, I felt so much better and had fun while doing it. But once I got pregnant with Torri, I decided to go into accounting as I am great with numbers. A logical explanation? Maybe not – but I did like working with numbers.

But now, I had a very important job, the most important ever, to help others feel comfortable in their own skin. Achieving my goal of weight loss has been the most challenging and fulfilling goal I have ever set for myself. I wanted others to believe, a "yes you can" philosophy.

As a trainer, and one who spent most of her life fat, my clients knew I could help them. They could learn from my life experiences. And it was more than teaching people how to weight train; I helped them be okay with who they were. I would not allow them to feel sorry for themselves. It may not have been tough love but I told them, "Tough, this is where you are today. Enjoy your journey because this will be the last weight journey you will have. This is a lifelong commitment." Every person needs to work out in some way or another – forever. I can show people how fun it is to stick to this commitment.

If my clients whined about how tough it would be to lose twenty pounds, I told them to quit their whining and be happy. They are not obese and they don't struggle to exercise or breathe. I would tell them to look at what I did, and they would shut up and suck it up.

I explained to people who are the size that I used to be that this is a journey – their journey – and that it would take time to start feeling better. Weight loss success is not instant. For the average person, it takes four-six weeks to actually begin to feel better. That's why it is important to stick with it and not give up. I even threatened to drive to some of my clients' homes and kick their butts. I've literally done this over a dozen times in the last two years. I mean business. Overweight and obese clients are my favorites because they work harder than all my other clients. They want to make me proud of them and I am.

My clients began to understand that weight is not a number on a scale. On my 5' 3-1/2" frame at 135 pounds, I am on the border of being overweight on a Body Mass Index (BMI) chart. A BMI chart takes into consideration a person's weight and height. It does not however take into consideration that muscle weighs more than fat. I do have a lot of muscle and my percentage fat continues to improve, but I have stayed the same weight on the scale for eight years. I have lost several sizes, but my weight has continued to stay the same. My "props" of five pounds of fat and five pounds of muscle are one of my best examples I use with my clients. The five pounds of fat appear to be double the size of the five pounds of muscle yet they weigh the same. I was checking out my BMI while waiting at my doctor's office and was surprised at what I saw.

Body Mass Index Table

	Normal					Overweight					Obese										Extreme Obesity															
BMI	19	20	21	22	23	24	25	26	27	28	29	30	31	32	33	34	35	36	37	38	39	40	41	42	43	44	45	46	47	48	49	50	51	52	53	54
Height (inches)												Body Weight (pounds)																								
58	91	96	100	105	110	115	119	124	129	134	138	143	148	153	158	162	167	172	177	181	186	191	196	201	205	210	215	220	224	229	234	239	244	248	253	258
59	94	99	104	109	114	119	124	128	133	138	143	148	153	158	163	168	173	178	183	188	193	198	203	208	212	217	222	227	232	237	242	247	252	257	262	267
60	97	102	107	112	118	123	128	133	138	143	148	153	158	163	168	174	179	184	189	194	199	204	209	215	220	225	230	235	240	245	250	255	261	266	271	276
61	100	106	111	116	122	127	132	137	143	148	153	158	164	169	174	180	185	190	195	201	206	211	217	222	227	232	238	243	248	254	259	264	269	275	280	285
62	104	109	115	120	126	131	136	142	147	153	158	164	169	175	180	186	191	196	202	207	213	218	224	229	235	240	246	251	256	262	267	273	278	284	289	295
63	107	113	118	124	130	135	141	146	152	158	163	169	175	180	186	191	197	203	208	214	220	225	231	237	242	248	254	259	265	270	278	282	287	293	299	304
64	110	116	122	128	134	140	145	151	157	163	169	174	180	186	192	197	204	209	215	221	227	232	238	244	250	256	262	267	273	279	285	291	296	302	308	314
65	114	120	126	132	138	144	150	156	162	168	174	180	186	192	198	204	210	216	222	228	234	240	246	252	258	264	270	276	282	288	294	300	306	312	318	324
66	118	124	130	136	142	148	155	161	167	173	179	186	192	198	204	210	216	223	229	235	241	247	253	260	266	272	278	284	291	297	303	309	315	322	328	334
67	121	127	134	140	146	153	159	166	172	178	185	191	198	204	211	217	223	230	236	242	249	255	261	268	274	280	287	293	299	306	312	319	325	331	338	344
68	125	131	138	144	151	158	164	171	177	184	190	197	203	210	216	223	230	236	243	249	256	262	269	276	282	289	295	302	308	315	322	328	335	341	348	354
69	128	135	142	149	155	162	169	176	182	189	196	203	209	216	223	230	236	243	250	257	263	270	277	284	291	297	304	311	318	324	331	338	345	351	358	365
70	132	139	146	153	160	167	174	181	188	195	202	209	216	222	229	236	243	250	257	264	271	278	285	292	299	306	313	320	327	334	341	348	355	362	369	376
71	136	143	150	157	165	172	179	186	193	200	208	215	222	229	236	243	250	257	265	272	279	286	293	301	308	315	322	329	338	343	351	358	365	372	379	386
72	140	147	154	162	169	177	184	191	199	206	213	221	228	235	242	250	258	265	272	279	287	294	302	309	316	324	331	338	346	353	361	368	375	383	390	397
73	144	151	159	166	174	182	189	197	204	212	219	227	235	242	250	257	265	272	280	288	295	302	310	318	325	333	340	348	355	363	371	378	386	393	401	408
74	148	155	163	171	179	186	194	202	210	218	225	233	241	249	256	264	272	280	287	295	303	311	319	326	334	342	350	358	365	373	381	389	396	404	412	420
75	152	160	168	176	184	192	200	208	216	224	232	240	248	256	264	272	279	287	295	303	311	319	327	335	343	351	359	367	375	383	391	399	407	415	423	431
76	156	164	172	180	189	197	205	213	221	230	238	246	254	263	271	279	287	295	304	312	320	328	336	344	353	361	369	377	385	394	402	410	418	426	435	443

Source: Adapted from Clinical Guidelines on the Identification, Evaluation, and Treatment of Overweight and Obesity in Adults: The Evidence Report

At my size I was a "24" – still within the normal range. But at 141 pounds I would be considered overweight. Needless to say I was ticked off and wanted to do an investigation. These numbers didn't seem right – or fair and I was ready to kick someone's ass over the chart. I reasoned that the BMI chart was probably invented by a man.

The BMI chart does not take into consideration the muscle mass – and muscle weighs more than fat as I just explained. Some idiot probably made this chart in the 1950's when women did not work as we do today. Today we work longer hours and work harder. I believe we do have more muscle than women had in the 1950's. We are not housewives, dressing in our pretty little dresses. We do everything a man does around the house. I cut my grass, power wash my house, and stain my deck. Heck, I've even built decks. It seemed to me that the BMI chart was outdated for these reasons alone. I did some investigating on who and when the BMI chart was invented.

Sure enough the chart was invented by a man – between 1830 and 1850. I really wasn't too upset with the guy. Times are far different from the 1800s when everyone was smaller. Actually, I was mad that we are still using BMI charts, which really compares a person's weight and height and does not take into consideration today's busy lifestyles. And that doesn't even include all the processed foods, chemical additives, pesticides or insecticides, and drugs used to promote animals growth, which I believe are reasons why we are all larger today. It's all about black-and-white numbers. It still sucks because this is the 21st century, not 1850.

My whole point is that goals should be attainable and sustainable – it's not about a number on a scale. If you can't attain a number on a scale, then it's not the number for you. If you can't sustain a number, it's not the number for you. I had to literally beat this point into some of my clients, some sustained major bruises. Not really.

As a trainer, I know my clients need to learn how to effectively work out with weights. I need to teach the importance of lifting heavy weights, even for women. The key to success is to lift heavy enough weights that the last two "reps" of every set are difficult to complete. Reps are repetitions, how many times you perform an exercise. For example, women should perform 12-20 repetitions per set and men 8-12 or 15. And I suggest doing that exercise three times to achieve maximum results.

Now comes the confusing part – in the literal sense. Many of my clients would perform the same exercise, time after time, in the gym. Maybe they were lazy or maybe they weren't remembering what was taught to them. Doing the same thing over and over again and expecting different results is the very definition of insanity. So, not only were these repetitious exercises boring, they were insane. And to top it all off, the muscles themselves got bored, too. I'll explain.

As I have said before in this book, people need to cause muscle confusion to consistently see results. They need to switch up their routine. For example, you should not perform "lat pull down" every time you train your lats. Lat is short for Latissimus Dorsi. These are the largest muscles in the entire upper body. They extend from behind each armpit to the middle of the lower back. There are tons of exercises to train your lats and each exercise hits your muscle a little different.

Here is a personal example from the "Lori file." When I was a teenager, I had a lawn business. In the beginning of the summer I would lose weight because of the strenuous exercise. The weight loss would then slow down toward the middle of the summer because my body got used to the movements and the muscles I used.

One of my clients bricks houses and buildings. It involves some very hard work. He goes up and down ladders and walks on scaffolds. The job includes lifting bricks, mixing mortar, and all kinds of strenuous work. He was chubby when he came to me, which may have seemed odd considering his work. He really never trained his legs a lot, often sitting on the scaffold when he worked. He had skinny legs, no butt and a large belly. He actually told me he did not need to exercise because he got his weight training at his job. Yeah, right. Six weeks later, following my training, he told me I was right. I love when men tell me I am right – because I usually am when it comes to training.

So, in this example, he trained all of his body parts, just once a week, and was able to lose six pounds in six weeks. His belly size went down, not from just core work, but also from working his large muscle groups, his legs, and butt. His lower back pain was gradually going away and he could stand longer at work.

Whether you are a guy or girl, working out effectively with weights will change your world. You must work each muscle group once a week, change up your routine to cause muscle confusion, lift heavy enough weights, stretch your body to help with flexibility, and do some cardio.

All of this will be explained later in this book. And if you follow these directions for six weeks, you will feel really good and understand what the heck I am talking about. For the first three-four weeks of the program, I want you to do the same exercises to become familiar with them and get you ready for the pain, errrrr, the fun. Then be ready to switch it up.

Chapter 12
The Birth of
Personal Trainer in a Box

I love my clients and my job as a personal trainer. I enjoyed training people that were truly interested in learning to become fit, and make a lasting impression on their lives. My clients have become my friends.

When my clients are not with me, I see them in the gym in a slight state of confusion. I think, hey, I have explained that exercise a lot and it hasn't sunk in. And I have also noticed a problem with their form – it isn't good. I know I am a good personal trainer but I shouldn't have to be in my clients' faces all of the time. Some clients would come in and be doing the same exercises without me.

So I began to type up explanations of how to set up the body, when to lift or lower, and where to feel the squeeze. I added how to breathe after a client asked if I would provide breathing instructions in a Word document. Another client asked if I could put my tips on cards for her so she could achieve maximum results. I did those tasks for them as an extra service. I was happy to do it. Still another client asked me if I could use pictures to go along with my tips. Okay, now something was beginning to take shape before my own eyes. I wish I could take credit for what happened next – but a lot had to do with client's requests.

Thus the birth of Personal Trainer in a Box, also known affectionately as "PT in a Box."

I had an idea for a similar product about a year earlier when studying to be a trainer. I even made little index cards. In fact, I still have them. I wanted to include some written instructions on how to effectively work out with weights, see positive results, achieve unbelievable energy, and feel better overall.

Here is how the program works – and why it will be the life-long program you will choose to be on. First, you will see and sustain your results. Second, you will feel so good that you will never give up again. Even if you "fall off the wagon" you will jump back on because you will know it does work. Physical fitness involves cardio vascular training, weight/resistance training, and flexibility/stretching training. PT in a Box has all three. You will also learn about sets, reps, and weight – and it is very important to pay close attention to all three while beginning. Circuit training and cardio training will also be explained.

You will learn to listen to your body, which is the key to any good workout. We are all at different fitness levels when we begin, so listening to your body is key. Important note: you should never feel pain while performing any exercise. If you do stop immediately and go see your doctor.

What about the muscles? I find this to be very important. I really did not understand my trainer's advice, which was to "get into the muscle." She said that, "Even with out weight you should be able to get inside the muscle and perform a move – and feel that muscle contract. " I didn't know what the heck she was talking about.

On every exercise I teach students to recognize "The Squeeze." This is what my trainer called getting inside the muscle and I explain when and where you should feel it. Many people, including me in the beginning, do not understand what each muscle does and why it is important. I do – and I'll tell you about that, too.

You will also learn how to breathe correctly, exhaling on the hard part. You will learn trainer tips such as "push with your heels" during a squat to make your time more efficient. These trainer tips are invaluable. When I learned how to perform exercises correctly with proper breathing, learned to stretch in between sets and followed expert tips, I saw the results I needed to continue on my journey.

You will learn about the theory of nutrition in "The Food Pyramid." I will explain later what I eat and why – and what results you can expect. Yep, everyone that does this program will see results and will become whatever size they want to become. For now, lets look at the basics of Personal Trainer In a Box.

You have just made a commitment to yourself to achieve lifelong health and well being with the Change Your World Fitness Workout. We make commitments everyday for others in life and follow through those commitments with tremendous focus. Why don't we follow through with commitments that are for our well being? We are always there for others, why won't we make a commitment for ourselves?

You might say that you don't have time to workout? The average American spends 4.5 hours a day watching TV. You might say I have to run my kids to dance or Karate. Who is going to run your kids to their events if you do not take care of yourself?

Physical fitness involves, Cardio Vascular Training, Weight/Resistance Training and Flexibility/Stretching. All of these need to be done properly to achieve a well tuned machine, your body. You only get one body in your lifetime, take care of it! Would you buy a brand new car and never change the oil? Of course not!

You could replace your car if it broke, you cannot replace your body. So take care of it. Part of that equation is exercise, the other part is diet. We will explain the exercise portion in detail and give you general guidelines on diet.

Working out with weights is the answer; it sculpts your body and increases your metabolism!

www.changeyourworldfitness.com

The Program & Workouts

THE PROGRAM

Let's get started on your journey to a healthy year! Change Your World Fitness.

To get started, you will select how many days a week you can devote to your program, the parts of the body you will be working out, the exercises you will perform and general recommendations about getting started.

If you are a beginner, we suggest that you perform the same exercises for 2-4 weeks to perfect those before moving onto other exercises. You will then need to perform the new exercises for 2-4 more weeks before moving onto different ones. Once you are through the entire tab of exercises, then switch it up weekly for a countless number of variations.

If you currently participate in an exercise program and feel you can handle the challenge of new exercises often, go for it! It's ever changing and you won't be bored. Once you perfect these, you can then move onto "Change Your World Fitness' "Hardbody" edition. This great mix of exercises builds muscle faster and keeps this program interesting.

Remember to read about each muscle on the muscle tab and warm up prior to working out. Become familiar with your muscles, by warming up before and stretching during and after every workout!

www.changeyourworldfitness.com

Circuit & Cardio/Interval Training

CIRCUIT TRAINING

You may decide to do these exercises with little or no rest between sets and exercises. This is called interval training, because you do not in rest in between sets while receiving benefits of aerobic/cardio training.

Circuit Training is great for those of you who are short on time. We would still like you to get your cardio in at least 3 days a week, but circuit training can provide Anaerobic (without oxygen) and Aerobic (with oxygen) benefits.

Why is this good? With little rest in between sets and exercises, your heart rate stays elevated and you burn more calories during that routine. We suggest buying and wearing a heart rate monitor during Circuit Training and Cardio Training to provide you with statistics regarding your training. The Heart Rate Monitor provides statistics such as time trained, calories burned and heart rate. It's a must have when you are committed to making a health change.

www.changeyourworldfitness.com

Circuit & Cardio/Interval Training

CARDIO

Working out with weights (or resistance training) is needed to Change Your World Fitness, but there's much more. **Cardio, Cardio, Cardio!!!!!**

We suggest that you do 30 minutes of cardio at LEAST 3 days a week. We would prefer if you did low to moderate cardio, such as walking the dog, going for a bike ride the other days of the week.

If you look at the new Food Pyramid, you will see that the steps in the pyramid are to let you know that, as important as the food you eat, exercise is important to your well being.

TIP – Remember strength training will sculpt your body and give you muscle definition, but cardio is needed to keep your most important muscle healthy, your heart! No one ever died from weak Triceps!!!

Your Heart Rate – We suggest talking to your physician before starting any exercise program and determining your target heart rate. A formula to talk over with your doctor is 220-your age and then you need to know the intensity. The intensity is a percentage of that number. Our intensity is based on our goals and needs. 50-80% intensity is a good place to discuss with your doctor.

www.changeyourworldfitness.com

Each exercise card really does not discuss the starting weight, repetitions or sets. Everyone beginning this program is at a different place, so a little trial and error in the beginning is necessary. The Muscle Group Tabs have some general guidelines for each group of muscles that will include free weights and machines.

Some advice, if you are using dumbbells, we suggest starting with 5 pounds. Get your form perfect before you advance to a heavier weight. If you are performing exercises on machines, start low and see how difficult that weight is for you. We will give you some weight guidelines on each Muscle Group Tab.

Once your form is perfect, remember the big goal-your last few reps should be hard to complete without sacrificing form. You will either have to go up in weight or repetitions to advance to the next level with your body (or both).

Sometimes we go up in weight, other times, we may go down in weight and up in repetitions. Success comes from switching things up often, so your body does not get used to any one routine. That's the key to **Change Your World Fitness Personal Trainer**, the combinations are endless.

www.changeyourworldfitness.com

The Right Weight, Reps & Sets.

REPETITIONS AND SETS

For beginners, we suggest two sets and 8-12 reps. Two sets will help you remember how to do the exercise. Remember, practice makes perfect. Eight to twelve repetitions will provide feedback the next day as to how those muscles feel.

Generally, women should perform 3 sets of 12-15 reps and Men should perform 3 sets of 8-12 reps. Women generally do less weight and higher reps to achieve the body they desire. The key is diversity and change! Women, do not be afraid of increasing weights. We do not have the testosterone to look like a man. We need to challenge our bodies. Keep your body wondering what you are going to do tomorrow!

www.changeyourworldfitness.com

What Benefits Can I Expect?

For most of us, losing weight is our goal. Muscle tissue burns more calories than fat does, even while your body is at rest. The more lean muscle you have, the better your metabolism works. If two women weigh the same amount, say 135 lbs and one has more muscle than the other, the one with more muscle will burn more calories even while sitting on a couch watching TV! We all lose muscle mass as we age and our metabolism slows down and weight gain begins. Turn back the clock and increase your metabolism.

The solution we have provided for you is weight training. When you do cardio, your metabolism increases, but only while you are doing your cardio. So, if you're on an elliptical machine for 30 minutes, your metabolism will increase, but only while you are on that machine. When you work out with weights, your metabolism will continue to rise. You can expect this increased metabolism for up to 48 hours. If you weight train every other day, your metabolism will continue to burn more calories!

www.changeyourworldfitness.com

What Benefits Can I Expect?

As personal trainers, we see people all the time in the gym regularly that complete demanding workouts, but get minimal results. Their bodies don't change. These people don't even question their workouts; they typically blame themselves for not working out hard enough or long enough. The problem is that a person may do adequate cardio and stretching, but does not perform weight training effectively.

Part of the problem, with women especially, are the negative images associated with weight training. Women think that they will get big and bulky. That won't happen!

Another problem is that people do not know how to effectively perform the exercise, stretch and switch it up often. That's why some people train with personal trainers. The #1 complaint from our clients is that once they come to the gym by themselves, they forget how we did the exercise. As well as what stretch is for that muscle group and what exercises to do next!

WE SOLVE ALL OF THAT WITH CHANGE YOUR WORLD FITNESS WORKOUT!

www.changeyourworldfitness.com

NUTRITION IS A BIG PART OF THE SUCCESS THAT YOU WILL EXPERIENCE.

Nutrition is essential to any new work-out routine. Your body needs fuel to power you through a good strength training routine. We recommend that you eat a small amount of protein and carbs, one to two hours before your work out. Never work-out on an empty stomach.

Here are a couple of guidelines to start.
1. Drink at least ½ your body weight in ounces of water!
2. Limit your sodium to fewer than 2,000 mg per day.
3. Memorize the Food Pyramid Chart!
4. Keep a food journal!
(this is essential to success)

a. Record everything you eat and drink.
b. Record the amount of foods.
c. Note the time of each meal and snack.
d. Rate your hunger before and after each meal.
e. Only eat until you are not hungry, never full.
f. Eat often, 5-6 times a day with smaller meals.
g. Prepare your meals ahead of time, and have them handy (in the fridge or freezer) for those crazy days!

www.changeyourworldfitness.com

Visit www.mypyramid.gov for all the facts on what you should be eating.

This website is an invaluable tool! www.mypyramid.gov explains how many fruits and vegetables, dairy, lean meats, complex carbohydrates and fats you should be eating per day. It also explains why you should be eating good carbs, lean meats, and good fats.

We are not nutritionists, but we can definitely vouch for www.mypyramid.gov.

Another good source of information is The American Diabetes Association. They have all kinds of healthy eating plans that fit the needs of anyone wanting to eat healthy.

We would like you to talk to a physician about your caloric needs. An active woman, who works out, should never eat less than 1,600 calories per day/ 2,000 for a man. We should never go below 1,200 calories, EVER! You need fuel for your body to work efficiently. It wasn't food that made you fat; it was the wrong food and lack of exercise. Use food as fuel and exercise to expend energy and you will feel much better.

www.changeyourworldfitness.com

WORKOUTS

The workouts are designed to fit anyone's schedule whether you train at a gym, home or while on business. The first step is deciding how many days a week you can devote to your health! Generally most people, especially beginners should train every other day or the 3X a week model. This will provide enough time in between for your muscles to recuperate.

Whatever your reasons are for how many days per week you devote to training, just make sure you stick to your plan. If you have a bad week, get right back into the gym. You are worth it! You only get one body in life, make sure yours is running at its optimal level.

Stick To It! You Are Worth It!
Write an appointment in your planner for you to workout. You make time for everyone else, why not you? How are you going to take care of everyone else if you don't take care of yourself first?

All of us lead such hectic lives. We run the kids to this sport, that activity, this event, you get the point. We will put everyone ahead of our needs. Then we are so stressed, our own families do not even want to be around us. Working out can relieve stress, make you proud of YOUR accomplishments, CHANGE your body, make you STRONG and all of this is for YOU. It is time for a healthy change. There are lots of gimmicks out there, the only difference is this one really WORKS. If you work out with weights and adhere to a cardio program you will see the CHANGES and so will everyone else.

www.changeyourworldfitness.com

WORKOUTS

EACH OF US IS AT A DIFFERENT STARTING POINT ON OUR ROAD TO PHYSICAL FITNESS.

BEGINNERS

Beginners should begin with the 3X week schedule and stick with the same cards for a few weeks to become familiar with each exercise and then move on. Master them and then you can switch it up.

When you feel comfortable and your form is accurate, then switch it up to other exercises until you again have great form. So, every few weeks you try new exercises, depending on the parts of the body you are training that day.

Don't Forget to Change It Up!
For intermediate or advanced clients, pick something new every week. It is the change in exercises that make your body melt away! You may stick to a routine for a week or two or switch it up all the time. As long as your form is great, you can switch it up often.

As trainers, we KNOW why our clients see results much sooner than beginners on their own. We watch our clients to ensure their form is proper, make sure they are breathing, push them hard through motivating them and CHANGE it up often! All of this will be taught to you throughout the process!

YOU CAN DO THIS AND YOU ARE GOING TO LOVE IT (AND YOUR NEW BODY)!
www.changeyourworldfitness.com

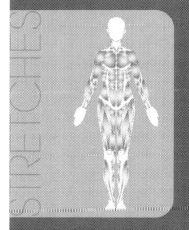

Stretching is a very important component to any exercise regime, yet often the most overlooked. Regular stretching reduces the risk if injury, relieves pain, improves and maintains flexibility, corrects poor posture and even helps counteract the effects of aging.

As we age, our bodies begin to dehydrate, making stretching even more important. Just as dehydration causes wrinkles on the exterior, it also affects the tissues on the interior. This causes our muscles, tendons and ligaments to dry out and tighten, therefore becoming leathery, over time, this causes the body to stiffen. Regular stretching will promote circulation of nutrients and water throughout the body.

EACH OF US IS AT A DIFFERENT STARTING POINT
ON OUR ROAD TO PHYSICAL FITNESS.

A stretch may target a muscle (or group of muscles) but you will feel its benefits throughout your body. As you go into a stretch, you will immediately feel the pull of your muscles upon your bones. Tendons connect muscles to bones and the pull of stretching can help the tendons "plump up",

therefore, helping to prevent injuries that often occur while working out.

While exercising, you should always stretch between sets and after working out. Hold each stretch for 20 seconds. You should begin your workout with a good warm-up routine.

ABOUT CARDIO AND TARGET HEART RATE

Cardio or aerobic exercise involves sustained, rhythmic exertion involving the large muscle groups such as legs, butt and back, which raises your heart rate enough so your cardiovascular system is exercised.

When you perform your cardio routine, you have to breathe harder and deeper, but should still be able to talk. Your metabolism increases while you are performing cardio. As soon as you are done, your metabolism returns back to normal (unlike weight training which raises your metabolism for up to 48 hours).

Here's a few reasons why cardio is so important:

- It's one way to burn calories and help you lose weight
- It makes your heart strong so that it doesn't have to work as hard to pump blood
- It increases your lung capacity
- It helps reduce risk of heart attack, high cholesterol, high blood pressure and diabetes
- It makes you feel good
- It helps you sleep better
- It helps reduce stress

Most of us should do our cardio routine for a minimum of 30 minutes and up to 90 minutes a day. Beginners should begin with 10-20 minutes. Check with your doctor before starting any exercise program and to find out your target heart rate!

www.changeyourworldfitness.com

SELECTION OF THE TYPE OF CARDIO

There are so many types of cardio; Walking, jogging, stair climber, elliptical trainer, studio cycling, jump roping, aerobic kickboxing, step aerobics, cross country skiing, mountain biking, rowing, inline skating and many more that will raise your heart rate.

Find what you like to do and get in your zone and go. The beginning is the hardest, be persistent and never give up. Some people like to do group classes, others like their favorite songs on their iPod and they get into their zone and go, others like to chit chat or watch TV. Whatever you need to do, get it done!

Interval training is an excellent way to train your cardio system. Going faster and then slower are really good ways to increase your cardio system. The jog/walk systems work well or just go faster and then recover on any cardio equipment.

Get a heart rate monitor! It will monitor your heart rate throughout your workout via a transmitter worn around your chest and a watch on your wrist.

With the talk test you should be able to carry on a conversation during your workout. If you are breathless, or can't talk, you're working too hard! Slow down. Also, keep in mind that dizziness and lightheadedness is not a good sign. If you experience this, you are overexerting yourself and should stop!

Try our combos in the next four cards of 15 minute bike, 15 minutes treadmill and 15 minutes elliptical for a great workout.

www.changeyourworldfitness.com

So now you have the gist of the program. I emphasize here and will continue to emphasize that it is really important to go talk to your doctor before beginning any workout routine, just to be on the safe side. This is especially true if you have any conditions such as high blood pressure, diabetes etc.

I am going to talk more in depth about what to eat and why later on. But in the next chapter, you will learn your new workout routine. All you need is weights, heavy enough to be difficult, a ball, and a mat. This is going to change your world.

Exercise Literally Makes You Younger!!!!!

It's a well known and documented fact that exercise literally makes you younger. Researchers recently discovered that a certain type of DNA strand called a "telemore," known to shorten as you age, actually gets longer the more active you are. In addition, exercise not only helps you look better, it makes you feel better – by reducing stress and elevating endorphins.

Chapter 13
The Two-Week Workout

Here is a two-week workout to give you a taste of how and why this will be the LAST fitness program you will ever be on for the rest of your life.

You will perform these exercises and repeat those same exercises for the first two-three weeks. As beginners, repeating exercises ensures you have a better understanding of the move. And it will give your body a chance to learn the move, become stronger, and then move on. In the future, you will be constantly switching up your routine to cause muscle confusion so that you never plateau. Go to our website www.changeyourworldfitness.com and get our full version of Personal Trainer in a Box. Put coupon code Thefatprincessnomore for 20% off the product.

Personal Trainer in a Box comes with over 124 exercises and 20 stretches. Over 87% of the exercises you can do from home. As you become more secure, I suggest joining a gym or buying a small home gym. I bought a great home gym.

My three favorite home gyms which I own or use at my clients homes are:

- Nautilus, with a Smith Machine
- The Total Gym
- Bioforce

Both the Total Gym and Bioforce can be purchased online, go to www.fitnessquest.com for all the details.

Overview for the next 2-3 weeks

Day One *(approximate time 30-45 minutes)*
Chest   2 exercises
Biceps   2 exercises

Triceps	2 exercises
Abs	2 exercises

Note: You will also stretch each muscle group between your sets.

Day Two *(approximate time 30-45 minutes)*

Thighs and Quads	2 exercises
Hamstrings	2 exercises
Glutes	2 exercises
Calves	1 exercise
Abs	2 exercises

Note: You will also stretch each muscle group between your sets.

Day Three *(approximate time 20-30 minutes)*

Back	2 exercises
Shoulders	2 exercises
Abs	2 exercises

Note: You will also stretch each muscle group between your sets.

Hey, did you notice you do abs every day you work out with weights? That is because your core is so important to your general health and a healthy lower back.

Here are some things that you should decide to do. Keep in mind that cardio must be completed, but your cardio is going to depend on what you have access to at home or gym.

You can use an elliptical, bike, stepper, treadmill, or walk. It's really up to you. During week one and two, plan on spending 20 extra minutes immediately following your weight training. After that, work up to 30-45 minutes on cardio.

I suggest a heart rate monitor – and make sure you can hold a conversation while performing your cardio. If you can't talk, then slow it down. This journey is not a sprint; it's a marathon, slow and steady.

I prefer to do my cardio immediately following my weight training. Why? Because after lifting weights, I use up all my stored energy. I go straight to do my cardio after lifting weights I am burning fat! If you desire to lose weight, this will make a huge difference. Plus, I seem to loosen up my muscles when performing cardio immediately following my workout.

An example workout of cardio:

0-5 minute,	
a steady stroll, say	2 MPH
6-7 Minute	2.5 MPH
7-8 Minute	2.8 MPH
8-9 Minute	2.6 MPH
9-10 Minute	2.9 MPH
10-12 Minute	3.0 MPH
12-14 Minute	2.8 MPH
14-16 Minute	2.5 MPH
16-18 Minute	2.4 MPH
18-20 Minute	2.0 MPH

If you do not know how fast you are going, here is a key: just go faster and slower every minute or two. This type of cardio training really helps your endurance to continue cardio, seeing progress quickly. These MPH are general guidelines, you may have to go slower or faster depending on your fitness level. It's time to interject one of my important reminders: Listen to your body. It is all about you!

As soon as you master 20 minutes of cardio, step it up to 30-45 minutes of cardio. Having a healthy heart will allow you to push a little harder down the road. If you can't do your cardio after weight training, because of time restraints or you don't yet have enough energy, it's okay to split them up. The biggest factor is to get it done. I sometimes do cardio on my days off from weight training.

Breathing and its "negatives" are very important to read on each exercise. You will learn to exhale on the hard part or the force phase of the exercise and you will perform that in one count. One count means on the way up you will count to one. You will inhale on the part that you resist gravity and you will count to two during this part of the exercise.

It is really important to breathe correctly, especially paying attention to resist gravity. You should not let the weight drop. Why? Because it is resisting gravity that builds your muscles, even releasing weights. And remember to read everything about that particular exercise before you begin.

The weight, reps, and sets are merely guidelines. Please listen to your body and adjust. Some exercises may be harder for you in the beginning. Read the "At Home" section to ensure you are performing each exercise correctly – without a workout bench or other equipment.

Your stretching must be completed between each set. You will do a set of the exercise, then stretch that muscle, do a set of the exercise, stretch and so on. Stretching in between sets is essential to building long, lean muscles, help prevent injury, increase muscle-tendon flexibility, enhance performance, improve range of motion, increase good sleep, alleviate muscle soreness, enhance well-being, decrease low-back pain, and help with post exercise cool down. Whew. Do you have enough reasons to stretch? I think so.

Important note: Always warm up before beginning your weight training. Five-to-ten minutes of cardio or some type of total body aerobic exercise works well.

Let's Get Started
Day One Workout: Biceps, Triceps, Chest

Biceps – Biceps really help shape the upper arm. Nice, toned biceps helps to contour your upper body.

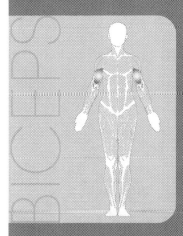

The *biceps* are among the most famous of all the muscles in the body. The *biceps brachii* is Latin for "two headed (muscle) of the arm" and is located on the upper arm. These two heads are called the: *Long Head* (attaches to the scapula) and the *Short Head* (attaches to the humerous). The primary function of the biceps is to flex the elbow and rotate the forearm. The Biceps muscle accounts for 1/3 of the overall mass of the upper arm.

www.changeyourworldfitness.com

EACH OF US IS AT A DIFFERENT STARTING POINT ON OUR ROAD TO PHYSICAL FITNESS.

Weight, Reps and Sets

Generally for our bicep muscle we will begin at certain weights depending on the exercise. Here are some general guidelines to follow.

	Dumbbells	Barbells*	Machine	Reps/Sets
Women	5-10lb	20lb	10-30lb	12-15/3 Sets
Men	5-20lb	20lb-30lb	20-40lb	8-12/3 Sets

*The barbell weight may be just the bar alone; some bars weigh 45lbs without weight. Beginners should perform one or two sets and generally 8-12 repetitions within the set.

www.changeyourworldfitness.com

These are general guidelines. Some of you will begin with lighter weight and some of you will begin with heavier weight. Listen to your body and remember, your last two reps must be harder to complete.

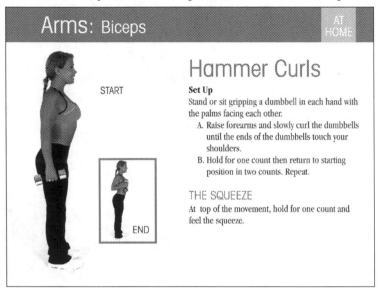

Arms: Biceps

AT HOME

Hammer Curls

Set Up

Stand or sit gripping a dumbbell in each hand with the palms facing each other.

   A. Raise forearms and slowly curl the dumbbells until the ends of the dumbbells touch your shoulders.

   B. Hold for one count then return to starting position in two counts. Repeat.

THE SQUEEZE

At top of the movement, hold for one count and feel the squeeze.

TIPS

- Keep elbows close to your body, only moving arm from elbow to wrist.
- Relax your hands.
- Do not rotate your wrists while curling.
- Proper technique can be achieved by using mirrors to check your form.
- Use slow and controlled movements.
- Contract your abs throughout the entire movement.

BREATHING & THE NEGATIVES

- Exhale as you lift the weights up, during the force phase of the exercise.
- Inhale during the resistance or the way down.
- On the way down, resist letting gravity take over. Resisting gravity is an important part of the exercise and really strengthens the muscle.
- One count on the way up and two counts on the way down, resisting gravity.

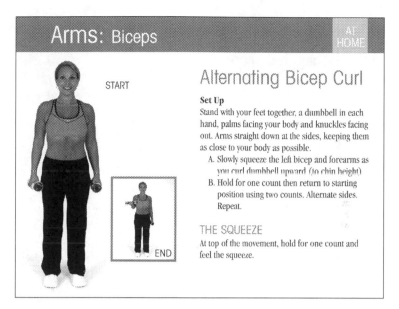

AT HOME

START

END

Alternating Bicep Curl

Set Up

Stand with your feet together, a dumbbell in each hand, palms facing your body and knuckles facing out. Arms straight down at the sides, keeping them as close to your body as possible.

A. Slowly squeeze the left bicep and forearms as you curl dumbbell upward (to chin height)

B. Hold for one count then return to starting position using two counts. Alternate sides. Repeat.

THE SQUEEZE

At top of the movement, hold for one count and feel the squeeze.

TIPS

- Relax your hands.
- Proper technique can be achieved by using mirrors to check your form.
- Use slow and controlled movements.
- Contract your abs throughout the entire movement.

BREATHING & THE NEGATIVES

- Exhale as you lift the weights up, during the force phase of the exercise.
- Inhale during the resistance or the way down.
- On the way down, resist letting gravity take over. Resisting gravity is an important part of the exercise and really strengthens the muscle.
- One count on the way up and two counts on the way down, resisting gravity.

Triceps – Triceps are very weak on most women, and that is why the guidelines say begin at three pounds, which is sometimes necessary. That's okay – the first few weeks you will see huge progress.

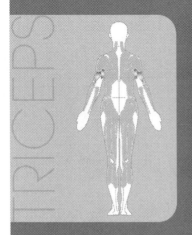

The triceps muscle runs along the back sides (posterior) of your upper arm. The triceps brachii is Latin for "three headed" (reflecting the three parts of the muscle).

The triceps brachii has three heads which connect the humerous and scapula to the forearm bone (ulna). These three heads are called the: Lateral head- (back of the humorous); Medial Head- (middle of humorous); Long Head- (bottom side of humorous).

The primary function of the triceps is to extend the elbow (or straighten the arm). The triceps muscle accounts for 2/3 of the overall mass of the upper arm.

www.changeyourworldfitness.com

EACH OF US IS AT A DIFFERENT STARTING POINT
ON OUR ROAD TO PHYSICAL FITNESS.

Weight, Reps and Sets

Generally for our triceps muscle we will begin at
certain weights depending on the exercise.
Here are some general guidelines to follow.

	Dumbbells	Barbells*	Machine	Reps/Sets
Women	3-10lb	20lb	10-40lb	12-15/3 Sets
Men	10-20lb	20lb-30lb	20-60lb	8-12/3 Sets

*The barbell weight may be just the bar alone; some bars weigh 45lbs without weight.
Beginners should perform one or two sets and generally 8-12 repetitions within the set.

www.changeyourworldfitness.com

These are general guidelines. Some of you will begin with lighter weight and some of you will begin with heavier weight. Listen to your body and remember, your last two reps must be harder to complete.

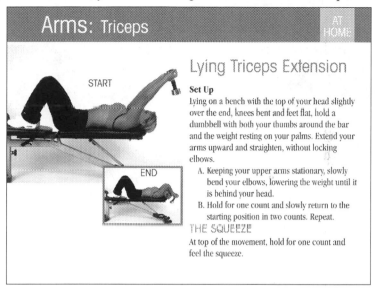

Arms: Triceps

AT HOME

Lying Triceps Extension

Set Up
lying on a bench with the top of your head slightly over the end, knees bent and feet flat, hold a dumbbell with both your thumbs around the bar and the weight resting on your palms. Extend your arms upward and straighten, without locking elbows.

A. Keeping your upper arms stationary, slowly bend your elbows, lowering the weight until it is behind your head.

B. Hold for one count and slowly return to the starting position in two counts. Repeat.

THE SQUEEZE
At top of the movement, hold for one count and feel the squeeze.

TIPS
- To ease back strain, lift your legs, pulling knees toward chest and cross your ankles.
- Use slow and controlled movements.
- Proper technique can be achieved by using mirrors to check your form.
- Contract your abs throughout the entire movement.

AT HOME
Do this at home using dumbbells, a bench, or the floor, or exercise ball.

BREATHING & THE NEGATIVES
- Exhale as you lift the weights up, during the force phase of the exercise.
- Inhale during the resistance or the way down.
- On the way down, resist letting gravity take over. Resisting gravity is an important part of the exercise and really strengthens the muscle.
- One count on the way up and two counts on the way down, resisting gravity.

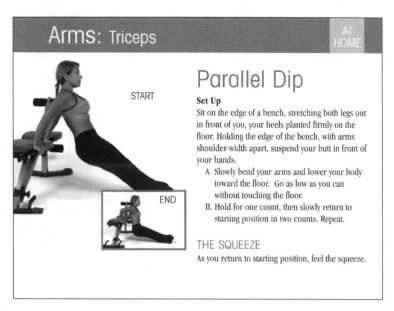

Parallel Dip

Set Up

Sit on the edge of a bench, stretching both legs out in front of you, your heels planted firmly on the floor. Holding the edge of the bench, with arms shoulder-width apart, suspend your butt in front of your hands.

A. Slowly bend your arms and lower your body toward the floor. Go as low as you can without touching the floor.

B. Hold for one count, then slowly return to starting position in two counts. Repeat.

START

END

THE SQUEEZE

As you return to starting position, feel the squeeze.

TIPS

- Do not lock your elbows on the upward movement.
- Use slow and controlled movements.
- Proper technique can be achieved by using mirrors to check your form.
- Contract your abs throughout entire movement.

AT HOME

Do this at home using a bench or stable chair. Beginners should bend your knees, so your feet are under your knees. Use your leg power to help you perform this.

BREATHING & THE NEGATIVES

- Exhale as you lift your body up, during the force phase of the exercise.
- Inhale during the resistance or the way down.
- On the way down, resist letting gravity take over. Resisting gravity is an important part of the exercise and really strengthens the muscle.
- One count on the way up and two counts on the way down, resisting gravity.

ATM

Chest – Ladies, we need to work out the chest. It will help defy gravity. Guys, this will create a balanced body and will help create a more V shaped upper body.

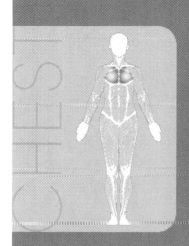

Your chest muscles are called *pectorals* (or *pecs* in the gym). The pecs are made of two muscles and they are called: *the Pectoralis Major*, the largest of the two. A thick triangular muscle spanning most of the collarbone, breastbone and connecting to the upper arm. *The Pectoris Minor* muscle, smaller and located beneath it's counterpart.

The primary function of the pectorals is to bring the arms toward the chest and medial rotation of the arm.

www.changeyourworldfitness.com

EACH OF US IS AT A DIFFERENT STARTING POINT ON OUR ROAD TO PHYSICAL FITNESS.

Weight, Reps and Sets

Generally for our chest muscle we will begin at certain weights depending on the exercise. Here are some guidelines to follow.

	Dumbbells	Barbells*	Machine	Reps/Sets
Women	5-10lb	20lb	10-20lb	12-15/3 Sets
Men	10-20lb	30lb	20-60lb	8-12/3 Sets

*The barbell weight may be just the bar alone; some bars weigh 45lbs without weight. Beginners should perform one or two sets and generally 8-12 repetitions within the set.

www.changeyourworldfitness.com

These are general guidelines. Some of you will begin with lighter weight and some of you will begin with heavier weight. Listen to your body and remember, your last two reps must be harder to complete.

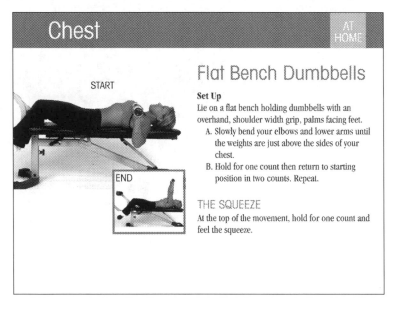

Chest AT HOME

Flat Bench Dumbbells

START

Set Up
Lie on a flat bench holding dumbbells with an overhand, shoulder width grip, palms facing feet.
A. Slowly bend your elbows and lower arms until the weights are just above the sides of your chest.
B. Hold for one count then return to starting position in two counts. Repeat.

END

THE SQUEEZE
At the top of the movement, hold for one count and feel the squeeze.

TIPS

- To ease back strain, lift your legs, pulling knees toward chest and cross your ankles.
- Proper technique can be achieved by using mirrors to check your form.
- Use slow and controlled movements.
- Contract your abs throughout the entire movement.

AT HOME

Do this at home using dumbbells, a bench, exercise ball, or floor if needed. The floor will prevent the full range of motion.

BREATHING & THE NEGATIVES

- Exhale as you lift the weights up, during the force phase of the exercise.
- Inhale during the resistance or the way down.
- On the way down, resist letting gravity take over. Resisting gravity is an important part of the exercise and really strengthens the muscle.
- One count on the way up and two counts on the way down, resisting gravity.

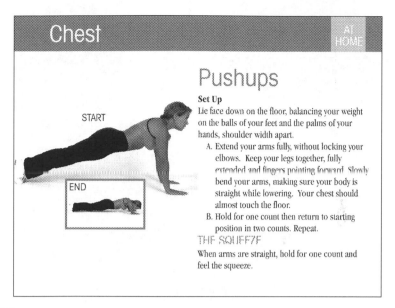

Chest

Pushups

Set Up

Lie face down on the floor, balancing your weight on the balls of your feet and the palms of your hands, shoulder width apart.

A. Extend your arms fully, without locking your elbows. Keep your legs together, fully extended and fingers pointing forward. Slowly bend your arms, making sure your body is straight while lowering. Your chest should almost touch the floor.

B. Hold for one count then return to starting position in two counts. Repeat.

THE SQUEEZE

When arms are straight, hold for one count and feel the squeeze.

START

END

TIPS

- If you are unable to do full pushups, do these on your knees instead of toes.
- On the upward motion, your legs, back and neck should be in one straight line.
- Proper technique can be achieved by using mirrors to check your form.
- Use slow and controlled movements.
- Contract your abs throughout the entire movement.

AT HOME

Do this at home or anywhere.

BREATHING & THE NEGATIVES

- Exhale as you push yourself up, during the force phase of the exercise.
- Inhale during the resistance or the way down.
- On the way down, resist letting gravity take over. Resisting gravity is an important part of the exercise and really strengthens the muscle.
- One count on the way up and two counts on the way down, resisting gravity.

Abs – Abs are my favorite! Your core is so important and you will see many changes in your abs. If you experience any lower back pain, bend your knees, bringing your knees into your chest. If your lower back still hurts or is strained, stop those exercises immediately and talk to your doctor.

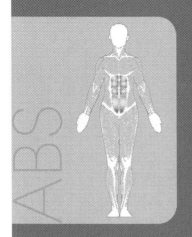

The *abdominal muscles* (or abs in the gym) consist of several muscle groups.

Rectus abdominus- the most notable of the *ab* muscles, start near the middle of the sternum and run vertically below the navel (this muscle gives you the "washboard" look).

Transversus abdominus- This muscle group is beneath the *rectus abdominus*. They compress and support the internal organs.

The *obliques*- The *external* and *internal obliques* extend up and down your sides. Trims the waist.

The primary function of the *abdominal muscles* is to stabilize the spine, protect internal organs, rotate and bend your body.

www.changeyourworldfitness.com

EACH OF US IS AT A DIFFERENT STARTING POINT ON OUR ROAD TO PHYSICAL FITNESS.

Weight, Reps and Sets
Generally for our ab muscle we will begin at certain weights depending on the exercise. Here are some guidelines to follow.

	Dumbbells	Barbells*	Machine	Reps/Sets
Women	5-10lb	N/A	10-45lb	12-15/3 Sets
Men	5-10lb	N/A	10-50lb	8-12/3 Sets

*The barbell weight may be just the bar alone; some bars weigh 45lbs without weight. Beginners should perform one or two sets and generally 8-12 repetitions within the set.

www.changeyourworldfitness.com

These are general guidelines. Some of you will begin with lighter weight and some of you will begin with heavier weight. Listen to your body and remember, your last two reps must be harder to complete.

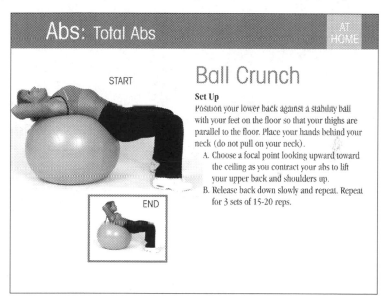

AT HOME

START

Ball Crunch

Set Up

Position your lower back against a stability ball with your feet on the floor so that your thighs are parallel to the floor. Place your hands behind your neck (do not pull on your neck).

A. Choose a focal point looking upward toward the ceiling as you contract your abs to lift your upper back and shoulders up.

B. Release back down slowly and repeat. Repeat for 3 sets of 15-20 reps.

END

TIPS

- Use slow and controlled movements.
- Proper technique can be achieved by using mirrors to check your form.
- Contract your abs throughout the entire movement.

AT HOME

Do this at home with an exercise ball.

BREATHING & THE NEGATIVES

- Exhale during the force phase of the exercise. Exhale when you lift your head off the ball.
- Inhale during the resistance as you lower back down to start.
- Resist letting gravity take over. Resisting gravity is an important part of the exercise and really strengthens the muscle.
- One count on the way up and two counts on the way down, resisting gravity.

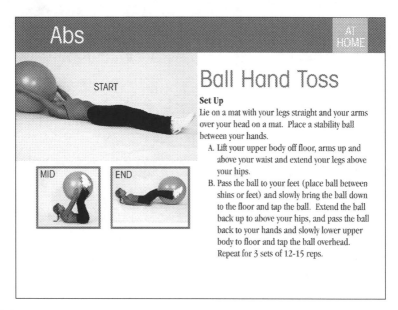

START

MID

END

Ball Hand Toss

Set Up

Lie on a mat with your legs straight and your arms over your head on a mat. Place a stability ball between your hands.

A. Lift your upper body off floor, arms up and above your waist and extend your legs above your hips.

B. Pass the ball to your feet (place ball between shins or feet) and slowly bring the ball down to the floor and tap the ball. Extend the ball back up to above your hips, and pass the ball back to your hands and slowly lower upper body to floor and tap the ball overhead. Repeat for 3 sets of 12-15 reps.

TIPS

- Gently touch the ball to the floor, no resting in between.
- If you experience lower back strain or pain, bend your knees and hold the ball with your knees instead of your toes.
- Use slow and controlled movements.
- Proper technique can be achieved by using mirrors to check your form.
- Contract your abs throughout the entire movement.

AT HOME

You can do this at home with a stability ball.

BREATHING & THE NEGATIVES

- Exhale during the force phase of the exercise. Exhale as contract your abs and lift your upper body up and pass ball to legs.
- Inhale during the resistance as you slowly return to start.
- Resist letting gravity take over. Resisting gravity is an important part of the exercise and really strengthens the muscle.
- One count on the way up and two counts on the way down, resisting gravity.

Day 2: Quads, Hamstrings, Glutes, Calves

Strong quads and thighs are important to both girls and guys. If soreness persists after your workout, sit in a warm tub or have your honey, give them a rub out.

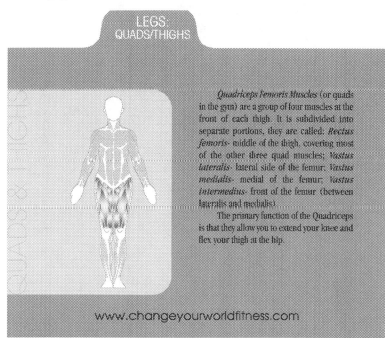

LEGS:
QUADS/THIGHS

Quadriceps Femoris Muscles (or quads in the gym) are a group of four muscles at the front of each thigh. It is subdivided into separate portions, they are called: *Rectus femoris*- middle of the thigh, covering most of the other three quad muscles; *Vastus lateralis*- lateral side of the femur; *Vastus medialis*- medial of the femur; *Vastus intermedius*- front of the femur (between lateralis and medialis).

The primary function of the Quadriceps is that they allow you to extend your knee and flex your thigh at the hip.

www.changeyourworldfitness.com

EACH OF US IS AT A DIFFERENT STARTING POINT
ON OUR ROAD TO PHYSICAL FITNESS.

Weight, Reps and Sets

Generally for our thigh/quad muscle we will begin at
certain weights depending on the exercise.
Here are some guidelines to follow.

	Dumbbells	Barbells*	Machine	Reps/Sets
Women	5-10lb	20lb	20-30lb	12-15/3 Sets
Men	20lb	30lb-40lb	30-60lb	8-12/3 Sets

*The barbell weight may be just the bar alone; some bars weigh 45lbs without weight.
Beginners should perform one or two sets and generally 8-12 repetitions within the set.

www.changeyourworldfitness.com

These are general guidelines. Some of you will begin with lighter weight and some of you will begin with heavier weight. Listen to your body and remember, your last two reps must be harder to complete.

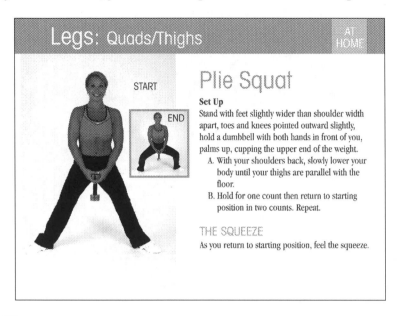

Legs: Quads/Thighs

AT HOME

START

END

Plie Squat

Set Up

Stand with feet slightly wider than shoulder width apart, toes and knees pointed outward slightly, hold a dumbbell with both hands in front of you, palms up, cupping the upper end of the weight.

    A. With your shoulders back, slowly lower your body until your thighs are parallel with the floor.

    B. Hold for one count then return to starting position in two counts. Repeat.

THE SQUEEZE

As you return to starting position, feel the squeeze.

TIPS

- If you do not feel an inner thigh stretch on the way down, you may need to widen your stance.
- Use slow and controlled movements.
- Proper technique can be achieved by using mirrors to check your form.
- Contract your abs throughout the entire movement.

BREATHING & THE NEGATIVES

- Exhale as you lift the weights up, during the force phase of the exercise.
- Inhale during the resistance or the way down.
- On the way down, resist letting gravity take over. Resisting gravity is an important part of the exercise and really strengthens the muscle.
- One count on the way up and two counts on the way down, resisting gravity.

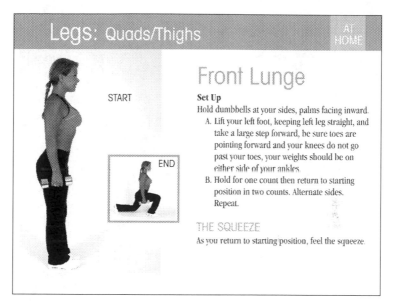

AT HOME

Front Lunge

START

END

Set Up

Hold dumbbells at your sides, palms facing inward.

A. Lift your left foot, keeping left leg straight, and take a large step forward, be sure toes are pointing forward and your knees do not go past your toes, your weights should be on either side of your ankles.

B. Hold for one count then return to starting position in two counts. Alternate sides. Repeat.

THE SQUEEZE

As you return to starting position, feel the squeeze.

TIPS

- Keep your chest lifted and shoulders back as you lunge forward.
- Your knee should not go past your toes.
- Use slow and controlled movements.
- Proper technique can be achieved by using mirrors to check your form.
- Contract your abs throughout the entire movement.

AT HOME

Do this at home using dumbbells or no weight at all.

BREATHING & THE NEGATIVES

- Exhale as you stand up, during the force phase of the exercise. Inhale during the resistance or the way down.
- Inhale during the resistance or the way down.
- On the way down, resist letting gravity take over. Resisting gravity is an important part of the exercise and really strengthens the muscle.
- One count on the way up and two counts on the way down, resisting gravity.

Legs: Hamstrings – The back of your legs are where your hamstrings are located. Important note: Make sure your hamstrings are warmed up before performing your hamstring exercise. Hamstrings are easily injured and take a long time to heal.

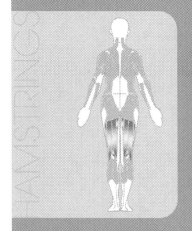

The *hamstrings* are a group of three muscles at the back of each thigh running from the knee to the hips. The word *ham* originally referred to the fat and muscle behind the knee. *String* refers to the tendons, and thus the hamstrings are stringlike tendons felt on either side of the back of the knee, the *long muscle*. The primary function of the hamstring is to allow you to bend your knee.

* Always warm up before exercising the hamstrings as they are the most commonly injured thigh muscles and are slow to heal.

www.changeyourworldfitness.com

EACH OF US IS AT A DIFFERENT STARTING POINT
ON OUR ROAD TO PHYSICAL FITNESS.

Weight, Reps and Sets

Generally for our hamstring muscle we will begin at certain weights depending on the exercise.
Here are some guidelines to follow.

	Dumbbells	Barbells*	Machine	Reps/Sets
Women	5-10lb	20-45lb	30-60lb	12-15/3 Sets
Men	10-20lb	45lb	40-70lb	8-12/3 Sets

*The barbell weight may be just the bar alone; some bars weigh 45lbs without weight.
Beginners should perform one or two sets and generally 8-12 repetitions within the set.

www.changeyourworldfitness.com

These are general guidelines. Some of you will begin with lighter weight and some of you will begin with heavier weight. Listen to your body and remember, your last two reps must be harder to complete.

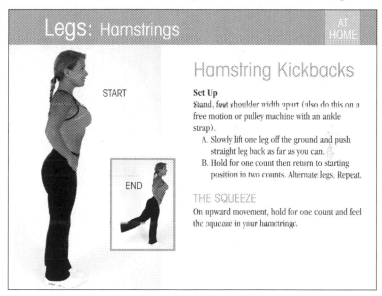

Legs: Hamstrings

Hamstring Kickbacks

START

END

Set Up
Stand, feet shoulder width apart (also do this on a free motion or pulley machine with an ankle strap).
  A. Slowly lift one leg off the ground and push straight leg back as far as you can.
  B. Hold for one count then return to starting position in two counts. Alternate legs. Repeat.

THE SQUEEZE
On upward movement, hold for one count and feel the squeeze in your hamstrings.

TIPS
- Stand up straight during movement.
- Bring leg back as far as possible without arching back.
- Use slow and controlled movements.
- Proper technique can be achieved by using mirrors to check your form.
- Contract your abs throughout the entire movement.

AT HOME
Do this exercise using ankle weights as you progress.

BREATHING & THE NEGATIVES
- Exhale as you lift leg up, during the force phase of the exercise.
- Inhale during the resistance or the way down.
- On the way down, resist letting gravity take over. Resisting gravity is an important part of the exercise and really strengthens the muscle.
- One count on the way up and two counts on the way down, resisting gravity.

Dumbbell Lying Hamstring Curl

START

END

Set Up

Lie face down on a bench, your knees just off the bench, position a dumbbell between your feet so the top of the weight is resting on your shoes. Grip the underside of the bench for support.

    A. Curl your ankles toward your butt while squeezing the weight between your feet.

    B. Hold for one count then return to starting position in two counts. Repeat.

THE SQUEEZE

At top of the movement. Hold for one count and feel the squeeze in your hamstrings.

TIPS

- Always keep a slight bend in your knees so you don't hyper-extend.
- Use slow and controlled movements.
- Proper technique can be achieved by using mirrors to check your form.
- Contract your abs throughout the entire movement.

AT HOME

Do this at home using dumbbells and bench, an aerobics bench, ottoman, or floor.

BREATHING & THE NEGATIVES

- Exhale as you lift the weights up, during the force phase of the exercise.
- Inhale during the resistance or the way down.
- On the way down, resist letting gravity take over. Resisting gravity is an important part of the exercise and really strengthens the muscle.
- One count on the way up and two counts on the way down, resisting gravity.

Glutes – Glutes make up the shape and appearance of your butt. I know this first hand, taking my flat butt that went out the sides creating saddlebags to my bootlicious butt today. When I stop by gym women say they love my butt. (In an admiring sort of way.) If you butt is too big, these exercises will make it smaller. If your butt is flat, you will be rounder and higher. Ad if you're a guy, we want you to have a nice butt don't you? So please work it out.

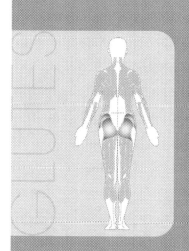

The *gluteal group* is composed of three separate muscles: the *gluteus maximus* (or *glutes* in the gym) is the largest and most superficial of the the *gluteal muscles*. It makes up a large portion of the shape and appearance of the buttocks.

The *gluteus minimus* – a smaller, deep seated muscle. The *gluteus medius*, one of the three gluteal muscles, is a broad, thick, radiating muscle, situated on the outer surface of the pelvis.

The primary function of the gluteal group is hip extension, as well as inward and outward rotation of the femur.

www.changeyourworldfitness.com

EACH OF US IS AT A DIFFERENT STARTING POINT ON OUR ROAD TO PHYSICAL FITNESS.

Weight, Reps and Sets

Generally for our glute/butt muscle we will begin at certain weights depending on the exercise. Here are some guidelines to follow.

	Dumbbells	Barbells*	Machine	Reps/Sets
Women	5-10lb	20-45lb	10-45lb	12-15/3 Sets
Men	10-20lb	45lb	40-70lb	8-12/3 Sets

*The barbell weight may be just the bar alone; some bars weigh 45lbs without weight. Beginners should perform one or two sets and generally 8-12 repetitions within the set.

www.changeyourworldfitness.com

These are general guidelines. Some of you will begin with lighter weight and some of you will begin with heavier weight. Listen to your body and remember, your last two reps must be harder to complete.

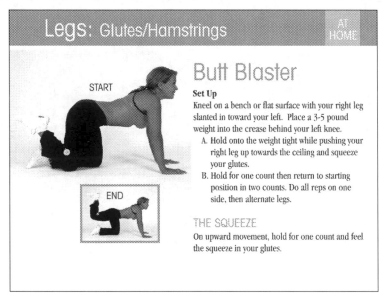

Legs: Glutes/Hamstrings — AT HOME

Butt Blaster

START

END

Set Up

Kneel on a bench or flat surface with your right leg slanted in toward your left. Place a 3-5 pound weight into the crease behind your left knee.

A. Hold onto the weight tight while pushing your right leg up towards the ceiling and squeeze your glutes.

B. Hold for one count then return to starting position in two counts. Do all reps on one side, then alternate legs.

THE SQUEEZE

On upward movement, hold for one count and feel the squeeze in your glutes.

TIPS

- Do not swing your leg.
- Use slow and controlled movements.
- Proper technique can be achieved by using mirrors to check your form.
- Contract your abs throughout the entire movement.

AT HOME

Do this at home with dumbbells or no weights.

BREATHING & THE NEGATIVES

- Exhale as you lift the weights up, during the force phase of the exercise.
- Inhale during the resistance or the way down.
- On the way down, resist letting gravity take over. Resisting gravity is an important part of the exercise and really strengthens the muscle.
- One count on the way up and two counts on the way down, resisting gravity.

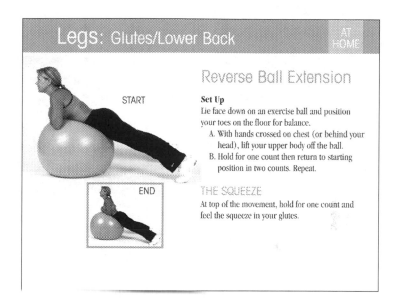

Legs: Glutes/Lower Back

AT HOME

Reverse Ball Extension

START

END

Set Up

Lie face down on an exercise ball and position your toes on the floor for balance.

A. With hands crossed on chest (or behind your head), lift your upper body off the ball.

B. Hold for one count then return to starting position in two counts. Repeat.

THE SQUEEZE

At top of the movement, hold for one count and feel the squeeze in your glutes.

TIPS

- It can be hard to balance the ball. Beginners should spread feet and legs wider for stability.
- Use slow and controlled movements.
- Proper technique can be achieved by using mirrors to check your form.
- Contract your abs throughout the entire movement.

BREATHING & THE NEGATIVES

- Exhale as you lift your body up, during the force phase of the exercise.
- Inhale during the resistance or the way down.
- On the way down, resist letting gravity take over. Resisting gravity is an important part of the exercise and really strengthens the muscle.
- One count on the way up and two counts on the way down, resisting gravity.

Calves – Calves need to be worked independently from your legs. They are often overlooked in other workout routines. When you feel a little burning sensation, do one or two more. That's it!

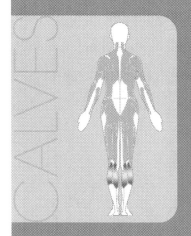

Calf muscles are hard to train, yet you don't need to spend a lot of time on them. The calf consists of two muscles, they are called: the *gastrocnemius*, this muscle has two heads that when fully developed appear diamond shaped. It attaches to the heel with the Achilles tendon; the *soleus*- this is a broad, flat muscle below the *gastrocnemius*.

The primary function of these muscles is to elevate the heel.

www.changeyourworldfitness.com

EACH OF US IS AT A DIFFERENT STARTING POINT
ON OUR ROAD TO PHYSICAL FITNESS.

Weight, Reps and Sets
Generally for our calf muscle we will begin at
certain weights depending on the exercise.
Here are some guidelines to follow.

	Dumbbells	Barbells*	Machine	Reps/Sets
Women	5-10lb	20-45lb	20-60lb	12-15/3 Sets
Men	10-20lb	45lb	40-70lb	8-12/3 Sets

*The barbell weight may be just the bar alone; some bars weigh 45lbs without weight.
Beginners should perform one or two sets and generally 8-12 repetitions within the set.

www.changeyourworldfitness.com

These are general guidelines. Some of you will begin with lighter weight and some of you will begin with heavier weight. Listen to your body and remember, your last two reps must be harder to complete.

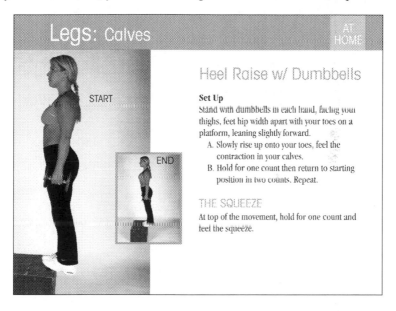

Legs: Calves

Heel Raise w/ Dumbbells

START

END

Set Up

Stand with dumbbells in each hand, facing your thighs, feet hip width apart with your toes on a platform, leaning slightly forward.

A. Slowly rise up onto your toes, feel the contraction in your calves.

B. Hold for one count then return to starting position in two counts. Repeat.

THE SQUEEZE

At top of the movement, hold for one count and feel the squeeze.

TIPS

- Keep your shoulders relaxed during movement.
- Use slow and controlled movements.
- Proper technique can be achieved by using mirrors to check your form.
- Contract your abs throughout the entire movement.

AT HOME

Do this at home using dumbbells and the bottom step of stairs.

BREATHING & THE NEGATIVES

- Exhale as you lift up, during the force phase of the exercise.
- Inhale during the resistance or the way down.
- On the way down, resist letting gravity take over. Resisting gravity is an important part of the exercise and really strengthens the muscle.
- One count on the way up and two counts on the way down, resisting gravity.

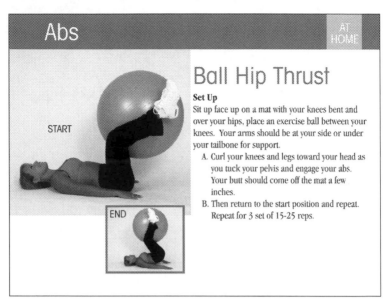

AT HOME

Ball Hip Thrust

Set Up

Sit up face up on a mat with your knees bent and over your hips, place an exercise ball between your knees. Your arms should be at your side or under your tailbone for support.

A. Curl your knees and legs toward your head as you tuck your pelvis and engage your abs. Your butt should come off the mat a few inches.

B. Then return to the start position and repeat. Repeat for 3 set of 15-25 reps.

START

END

TIPS

- Squeeze your knees together against the resistance ball to engage your inner thighs.
- Use slow and controlled movements.
- Proper technique can be achieved by using mirrors to check your form.
- Contract your abs throughout the entire movement.

AT HOME

Do this with an exercise ball. This is a small movement for beginners (1-2 inches to start).

BREATHING & THE NEGATIVES

- Exhale during the force phase of the exercise. Exhale when your legs curl towards your head.
- Inhale during the resistance as your legs go back to start.
- Resist letting gravity take over. Resisting gravity is an important part of the exercise and really strengthens the muscle.
- One count on the way out and two counts on the way down, resisting gravity.

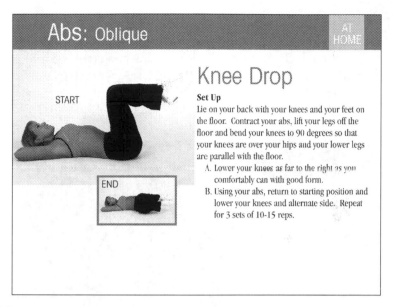

Knee Drop

START

END

Set Up

Lie on your back with your knees and your feet on the floor. Contract your abs, lift your legs off the floor and bend your knees to 90 degrees so that your knees are over your hips and your lower legs are parallel with the floor.

A. Lower your knees as far to the right as you comfortably can with good form.

B. Using your abs, return to starting position and lower your knees and alternate side. Repeat for 3 sets of 10-15 reps.

TIPS

- Keep your shoulders down and away from your ears.
- Keep your knees over your hips.
- Push your lower back into the floor.
- Use slow and controlled movements.
- Proper technique can be achieved by using mirrors to check your form.
- Contract your abs throughout the entire movement.

BREATHING & THE NEGATIVES

- Exhale during the force phase of the exercise. Exhale when you pull your legs back to start.
- Inhale during the resistance as your legs go down to the sides.
- Resist letting gravity take over. Resisting gravity is an important part of the exercise and really strengthens the muscle.
- One count on the way up and two counts on the way down, resisting gravity.

Day 3: Back, Shoulders and Abs

A healthy back is key to a long, healthy, happy life, both the upper and lower back. A slightly muscular back looks good on anyone, man or woman. It can give that nice V shape which makes the waist appear smaller.

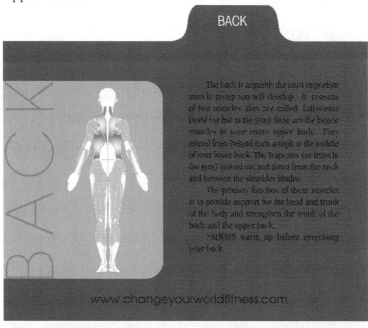

BACK

The back is arguably the most important muscle group you will develop. It consists of two muscles they are called: Latissimus Dorsi (or lats in the gym) these are the largest muscles in your entire upper body. They extend from behind each armpit to the middle of your lower back. The Trapezius (or traps in the gym) extend out and down from the neck and between the shoulder blades.

The primary function of these muscles is to provide support for the head and trunk of the body and strengthen the trunk of the body and the upper back.

*ALWAYS warm up before exercising your back.

www.changeyourworldfitness.com

EACH OF US IS AT A DIFFERENT STARTING POINT
ON OUR ROAD TO PHYSICAL FITNESS.

Weight, Reps and Sets

Generally for our back muscle we will begin at
certain weights depending on the exercise.
Here are some guidelines to follow.

	Dumbbells	Barbells*	Machine	Reps/Sets
Women	5-10lb	20lb	20-50lb	12-15/3 Sets
Men	20lb	30lb-40lb	30-60lb	8-12/3 Sets

* The barbell weight may be just the bar alone, some bars weigh 45lbs without weight.
Beginners should perform one or two sets and generally 8-12 repetitions within the set.

www.changeyourworldfitness.com

These are general guidelines. Some of you will begin with lighter weight and some of you will begin with heavier weight. Listen to your body and remember, your last two reps must be harder to complete.

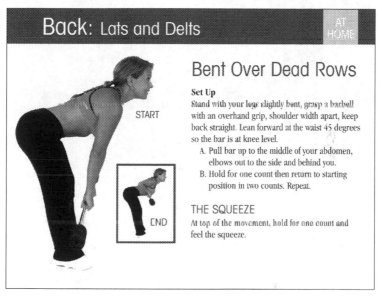

Back: Lats and Delts

AT HOME

Bent Over Dead Rows

Set Up

Stand with your legs slightly bent, grasp a barbell with an overhand grip, shoulder width apart, keep back straight. Lean forward at the waist 45 degrees so the bar is at knee level.

A. Pull bar up to the middle of your abdomen, elbows out to the side and behind you.

B. Hold for one count then return to starting position in two counts. Repeat.

THE SQUEEZE

At top of the movement, hold for one count and feel the squeeze.

START

END

TIPS

- Variation: one overhand grip and one underhand grip-hand wider than shoulder width apart.
- Proper technique can be achieved by using mirrors to check your form.
- Use slow and controlled movements.
- Contract your abs throughout the entire movement.

AT HOME

Do this at home using same movement with dumbbells.

BREATHING & THE NEGATIVES

- Exhale as you lift the weights up, during the force phase of the exercise.
- Inhale during the resistance or the way down.
- On the way down, resist letting gravity take over. Resisting gravity is an important part of the exercise and really strengthens the muscle.
- One count on the way up and two counts on the way down, resisting gravity.

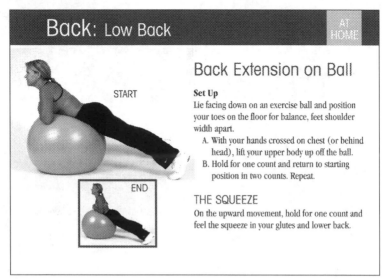

Back Extension on Ball

START

END

Set Up
Lie facing down on an exercise ball and position your toes on the floor for balance, feet shoulder width apart.
  A. With your hands crossed on chest (or behind head), lift your upper body up off the ball.
  B. Hold for one count and return to starting position in two counts. Repeat.

THE SQUEEZE
On the upward movement, hold for one count and feel the squeeze in your glutes and lower back.

TIPS
- Do not swing your body.
- If your lower back aches after workout, your form is wrong.
- Proper technique can be achieved by using mirrors to check your form.
- Use slow and controlled movements.
- Contract your abs throughout the entire movement.

AT HOME
Do this at home using an exercise ball.

BREATHING & THE NEGATIVES
- Exhale as you lift your body up, during the force phase of the exercise.
- Inhale during the resistance or the way down.
- On the way down, resist letting gravity take over. Resisting gravity is an important part of the exercise and really strengthens the muscle.
- One count on the way up and two counts on the way down, resisting gravity.

Shoulders – Shoulders need to be warmed up prior to working them out. One way to do this warm up is perform a couple of sets without weights. Shoulder injuries can be painful and often require surgery. As usual, go slow and listen to your body.

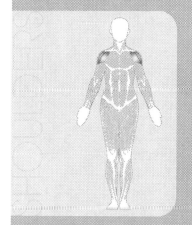

Your shoulder muscles are called *Deltoids* (or *delts* in the gym). Known also as *Deltoideus* in Greek meaning "triangle". A three-headed muscle that caps the shoulder. These three heads are called: *Anterior* (the front deltoid); *Lateral* (the middle deltoid); *Postorior* (the rear deltoid).

The primary function of the Deltoid muscle is to move the arm away from the body.

* ALWAYS warm up before exercising the Delts.

www.changeyourworldfitness.com

EACH OF US IS AT A DIFFERENT STARTING POINT
ON OUR ROAD TO PHYSICAL FITNESS.

Weight, Reps and Sets

Generally for our shoulder muscle we will begin at
certain weights depending on the exercise.
Here are some guidelines to follow.

	Dumbbells	Barbells*	Machine	Reps/Sets
Women	3-10lb	20lb	10-40lb	12-15/3 Sets
Men	10-20lb	20lb-50lb	20-60lb	8-12/3 Sets

*The barbell weight may be just the bar alone; some bars weigh 45lbs without weight. Beginners should perform one or two sets and generally 8-12 repetitions within the set.

www.changeyourworldfitness.com

These are general guidelines. Some of you will begin with lighter weight and some of you will begin with heavier weight. Listen to your body and remember, your last two reps must be harder to complete.

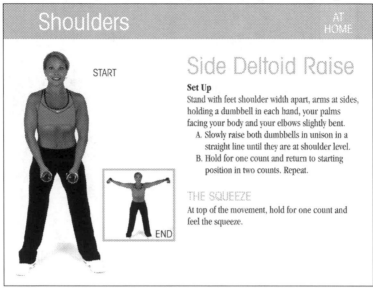

Shoulders AT HOME

Side Deltoid Raise

Set Up
Stand with feet shoulder width apart, arms at sides, holding a dumbbell in each hand, your palms facing your body and your elbows slightly bent.
A. Slowly raise both dumbbells in unison in a straight line until they are at shoulder level.
B. Hold for one count and return to starting position in two counts. Repeat.

THE SQUEEZE
At top of the movement, hold for one count and feel the squeeze.

TIPS
- Keep your shoulders down and back.
- Lead with your elbows and keep them slightly bent throughout the movement.
- Beginners should do one arm at a time.
- Use slow and controlled movements.
- Proper technique can be achieved by using mirrors to check your form.
- Contract your abs throughout entire movement.

BREATHING & THE NEGATIVES
- Exhale as you lift the weights up, during the force phase of the exercise.
- Inhale during the resistance or the way down.
- On the way down, resist letting gravity take over. Resisting gravity is an important part of the exercise and really strengthens the muscle.
- One count on the way up and two counts on the way down, resisting gravity.

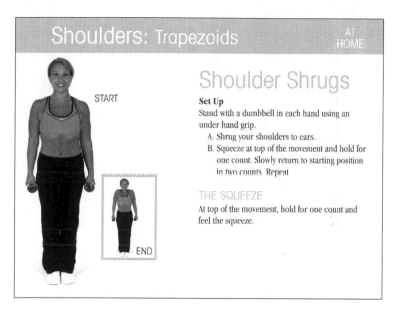

Shoulder Shrugs

Set Up

Stand with a dumbbell in each hand using an under hand grip.

A. Shrug your shoulders to ears.

B. Squeeze at top of the movement and hold for one count. Slowly return to starting position in two counts. Repeat

THE SQUEEZE

At top of the movement, hold for one count and feel the squeeze.

START

END

TIPS

- This is a great warm-up for your shoulders.
- Use slow and controlled movements.
- Proper technique can be achieved by using mirrors to check your form.
- Contract your abs throughout entire movement.

AT HOME

Do this exercise at home using dumbbells.

BREATHING & THE NEGATIVES

- Exhale as you shrug, during the force phase of the exercise.
- Inhale during the resistance or the way down.
- On the way down, resist letting gravity take over. Resisting gravity is an important part of the exercise and really strengthens the muscle.
- One count on the way up and two counts on the way down, resisting gravity.

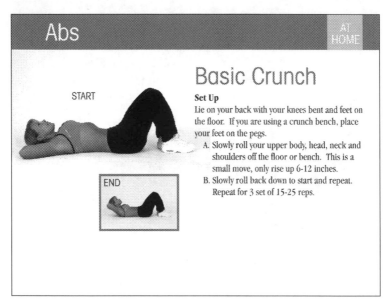

Abs ‎ AT HOME

Basic Crunch

START

END

Set Up

Lie on your back with your knees bent and feet on the floor. If you are using a crunch bench, place your feet on the pegs.

A. Slowly roll your upper body, head, neck and shoulders off the floor or bench. This is a small move, only rise up 6-12 inches.

B. Slowly roll back down to start and repeat. Repeat for 3 set of 15-25 reps.

TIPS

- Can be performed on a crunch machine at the gym. This provides a beginner with excellent form.
- Keep your elbows wide and out to the sides.
- As you lift up, your eyes should be focused on the ceiling.
- Use slow and controlled movements.
- Proper technique can be achieved by using mirrors to check your form.
- Contract your abs throughout the entire movement.

BREATHING & THE NEGATIVES

- Exhale during the force phase of the exercise. Exhale when you lift your head and shoulders up.
- Inhale during the resistance as you lower your head back to start.
- Resist letting gravity take over. Resisting gravity is an important part of the exercise and really strengthens the muscle.
- One count on the way up and two counts on the way down, resisting gravity.

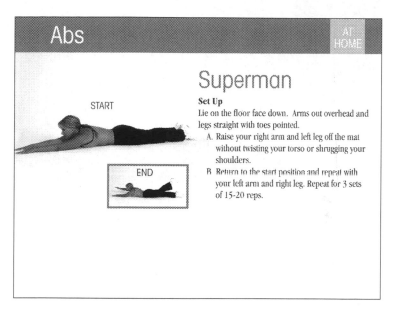

AT HOME

Superman

START

Set Up
Lie on the floor face down. Arms out overhead and legs straight with toes pointed.

A. Raise your right arm and left leg off the mat without twisting your torso or shrugging your shoulders.

END

B. Return to the start position and repeat with your left arm and right leg. Repeat for 3 sets of 15-20 reps.

TIPS

- Keep your shoulders down and relaxed.
- Lift your arm and leg as high as you can without sacrificing form.
- Keep the arm and leg straight as you lift.
- Use slow and controlled movements.
- Proper technique can be achieved by using mirrors to check your form.
- Contract your abs throughout the entire movement.

AT HOME

You can do this at home or anywhere.

BREATHING & THE NEGATIVES

- Exhale during the force phase of the exercise. Exhale as contract your abs and lift one arm and one leg.
- Inhale during the resistance as you slowly return to start.
- Resist letting gravity take over. Resisting gravity is an important part of the exercise and really strengthens the muscle.
- One count on the way up and two counts on the way down, resisting gravity.

You have just completed week one, great job.

Chapter 14
What Are You Eating
& Why?

Your health depends largely on what you eat. I classify health as your physical health, mental health, and emotional health. Now I am going to tell you what you should eat. Eating is part of the whole package – a key to making you feel better about yourself. If you want to be healthy in body, mind, and spirit, what you are eating is very important.

Yes, I could use the tired old cliché that people's lifestyles are busier – and there is less time to devote to taking care of one's self. We do a lot for everyone else, like our kids, and don't pay enough attention to our own physical and mental health. Knowing that should be scary. Why? Because who will take care of our families if we are not around? We must take care of ourselves first so that we can take care of everyone else in our lives. Fitness and nutrition go hand in hand.

I told you about Dad, having a brain stem stroke at age 51. He was three-and-a-half years from retirement and he had big plans. He would finally get to enjoy woodworking, or play tennis, or do whatever. His stress level would have dropped by 90 percent. But sadly, Dad never made it to that day. If only I could have taught him what I now know, maybe I could have saved him. But that is in the past now. I am dedicating my life to saving a lot of people who have their own future plans – right now.

Could you imagine, being gone from this Earth? Maybe I'm getting a little cerebral right now but it something that everyone should think about. A lot. How would your family and friends react? How would life go on for them? And what if all it took was a change in fitness and nutrition to help stick around longer for your family, friends, and you? I believe we would all make those changes – or should. Now I am asking you to change your eating habits to help you live a long, healthy life for you, your family, and loved ones.

This chapter will provide you with the basic knowledge you need to clean up you diet and enable you to fuel your muscles with good nutrition, so they are efficient. Many people I train have said, "I am seeing results, but my middle won't go down." I tell them it's their diet. Others have said, "I have big muscles, they just don't show up." I say, change your diet. Diet is amazing. Eating healthy will double your success on this program.

Healthy eating can create healthy body systems, which means what you eat can provide more nutrients to your body and your body will function optimally. This is the fastest route to improved health and well-being. What you eat can also help you fight diseases. And of course, what you eat can help you stay slim and young.

Here are some of my guidelines to try to begin having a cleaner diet.

Go Organic

Commercial farming uses chemicals to protect the crops or to promote growth in plants and animals. We are finding out that these chemicals are the cause of disease and some forms of cancer. I also have read reports that these chemicals may cause hyperactivity in children, infertility, mood swings, asthma, upset our hormonal balance, and other issues.

Of course I am not a nutritionist, but I do believe, eating a cleaner diet, free from chemicals is a good idea.

Here is a side note. As a Mom, I tried so hard to feed Torri perfectly. We ate very healthy, lots of low-fat dairy, lots and lots of chicken breast, lean red meats, veggies, fruits, and healthy oils. My daughter began puberty at age seven. At seven she also began to grow underarm hair – and emit the odor that goes with it. By eight, I had to shave her armpits and she began using deodorant. When she was eight, other "puberty changes" began happening to her. My point? I have read report after report on the Internet and I am convinced as a Mom that the chemicals to beef up the animals and the chemicals added to our dairy cows has not only made out kids bigger but it has brought them into puberty much faster.

When I was in school, not a lot of girls were overweight. But in the last few decades it's become an epidemic. When I was in school, it was not common to see a lot of large-breasted girls. Look around today.

Keep in mind that going organic is more expensive. Make sure you read the labels and look for descriptive text like "natural," "no hormones," or "no antibiotics."

Go to Your Local Farmers Market

In the "old days" we used to only eat what was in season. Freshness only lasted a short time. Now we are used to going to the grocery store and getting whatever we want. A bigger variety isn't necessarily a better variety. As much as you can, try to eat fruits and veggies in season. The nutrients are at their highest level.

Also, your local farmers markets are great place to buy in bulk. I love blueberries – can't get enough of them. I went blueberry picking earlier this summer and I brought home a whole bushel. I laid them out on a cookie sheet in one layer and put the cookie sheet in the freezer. I do this all of the time. Once frozen, I can put them in a freezer bag and they won't lose their shape or juices. Think ahead. Freezing is a great option to extend your fresh foods.

Ok, so what do I you eat to feed my muscles?

To get and maintain a healthy body you must nourish your body with the correct fuel. Like I said before, we all lead fast-paced, crazy lives and we do a lot for everyone else and not enough for ourselves. If we eat high quality food, especially lean protein and complex, and high fiber carbohydrates we will have the energy to dominate and thrive in our crazy, busy lives. And it will aid us to build muscle tissue and raise our metabolic rate. Speaking of metabolic rate, the higher it is, the more calories you burn while resting.

And before starting your new healthy eating plan, go to your local vitamin store and check into a good detoxification plan to enable your body to work more efficiently. Try this website, www.bodyandfitness.com. (Here is the link to the page I am talking about: www.bodyandfitness.com/Information/Health/detox.htm.)

Bodyandfitness.com has some unbelievable facts and brings up good points to why we do need to detoxify our body.

Boost my metabolism

1. Train your muscles at least three to four times a week. Training each muscle group once a week is all it takes. I use the three-day plan in my PT in a Box. Every other day gives my body a chance to have a rest. I do cardio almost every day, because I am type A personality and without cardio, I have ants in my pants and can't sit still.

2. Quit yo-yo dieting. Lack of food places your body in starvation mode and makes it harder to see progress. Fuel your body with the correct foods every 2-4 hours. Obviously you can learn from my mistakes and get off any and all diets, period. You need to eat every 2-4 hours, eat healthy foods, and stop being so strict on your choices. If a diet says you can't eat a food, throw that diet away. I starved for two years to take off 107 pounds. Knowing what I know now, I could have lost my weight healthier and faster. When you starve your body, your body goes into starvation mode, hanging on to everything you eat, storing it as fat. Why in the world would you want to do that? And then you get so hungry that you binge and eat double the calories you probably would have, had you just eaten healthy foods five-six times throughout your day.

3. Make good choices in what goes in your body. Think of your body like a Lamborghini car or whatever car you have longed for. Would you put bicycle tires on that car? Of course not. Would you maintain it properly? Of course you would. Fuel your body with good foods; you only get one body in your lifetime. And you can always replace an expensive car, you can't replace your body.

4. Get rid of simple carbs (white bread, sugary carbs) and replace them with complex carbs. A lot of weight loss diet plans push sugary supplements. I know if I eat a 100-calorie snack, I am never satisfied. So I avoid sugary carbs. The more I have, the more I crave and those are the days that I overeat. I went to a weight loss clinic many times and they sold me all these bars and snacks and gave me a sheet of when to eat what. It was a disaster. My supplements were supposed to last me two weeks and I devoured them in four days. They were like candy, and they had the sugar like candy. The more I ate, the more I wanted. If you want something sweet, have some fruit. At least you will get some great natural fiber, vitamins, and other good nutrition.

5. Keep meals small, eating 300-400 calories per meal. If you never want to binge again in your life, eat small meals spread throughout your day. I know you are going to tell me you don't have time. Make it! I cook a few healthy meals on Sunday and package them up for the week. I grill lots of chicken breast on Sundays too, and put them in individual baggies so I can grab and go. Usually by Wednesday or

Thursday I need to cook a few more meals and plan for the rest of my week. I also cut up fresh veggies and have them plentiful and ready. Have you ever tried fresh veggies and hummus? It's a great healthy snack. I even turned Jeff on to that one.

6. Eat five-six small meals a day. So, if you are eating 300-400 calorie meals you need to eat more often. And if you preplan, you won't have an issue. Your digestion is better when you eat smaller meals. Have you ever eaten a huge meal and really over-did it. How did you feel? Like crap? Don't do that to your body.

7. Eat protein and complex carbs at every meal (4-5 ounces of lean protein). Because I weight train, I do require a little more protein than I did before. I don't believe in the fad diets which are high in protein. Any diet that causes you to gain weight back while eating normally is bad. These fad diets will aid you to lose weight, but again, if you can't eat like that forever, then it is not good for you. If a diet excludes healthy foods, than it is not good for you.

8. Consume the good oils especially flax seed oil. Olive oil, flax seed oil, and fish oils are all essential to our new healthy body. In fact, essential good oils and fats can lower your bad cholesterol, increase your good cholesterol, lower your blood pressure, lower your risk of stroke, decrease your risk of macular degeneration, and reduce risk of Alzheimer's and Dementia. And you will experience better skin, improvements in arthritis, and better results for weight loss.

9. Make sure to hydrate your body with at least half your body weight in ounces of water. Drinking water enhances weight loss, helps with common ailments such as headaches, fatigue, and back pain – which may be the cause of dehydration. Drinking water can reduce hunger, often hunger pangs are often mistaken for the need for hydration. Drinking water can make you look younger. It plumps and radiates your skin. I know if I am dehydrated, my lines between my eyebrows get deeper and more noticeable. It's a sign to tell me to get some water. Listen to your body, it tells you things that you need. Do you want to know if you are drinking enough water, check your urine? If it is bright yellow it could mean you are dehydrated. If your mouth is dry or you feel dizzy, you really need water, fast.

10. Supplement with a great quality vitamin. I eat pretty healthy for sure but even now I take a multivitamin. When I had my plastic surgery, my doctor said I needed to get on a good multivitamin, maybe a prenatal. I said, "Hey I eat out of all the food groups and I am young and healthy." He convinced me. I take a good prenatal vitamin every day. (Make sure to tell your husband and family and friends why you are taking it, no need to falsely alarm them.) For guys, go to your local vitamin store and talk to one of the experts on which one is right for you.

11. Lift weights regularly. The benefits of weight training are so great. Although this chapter is mostly about food, I had to include weight training reminders in this chapter as well because nutrition and health go hand in hand.

12. Eat spicy healthy foods, and cinnamon. Love fiery peppers, curry, or hot sauce? In addition to making your taste buds sizzle, spicy foods can also deliver many health benefits. And they have antioxidant and anti-inflammatory properties that are beneficial to the body. Hot peppers can speed up metabolism and help the body burn calories faster. Other benefits may include help with types of cancers, Alzheimer's, mood, arthritis, heart health. Healthy spicy foods may boost your body's ability to dissolve blood clots and help with inflammatory issues in the heart.

13. Try to drink your coffee black. I sometimes use my vanilla protein powder in my coffee as a creamer to ensure my daily protein. I have stopped using sugar or sweetener. It does help cut down on my cravings for sweets if I don't have something sweet in my coffee. Second choice? Look for no sugar creamers. I would rather have no sugar than no fat. But again, sparingly, because all no sugar creamers mean is there is a sweetener in the product.

14. Dump the carbonated soft drinks. As a treat once in a while, I have a Diet Coke over some ice, and it's a treat. (Remember my "crash diet" involving Diet Coke and cigarettes?) You need to drink more water, less soda or pop.

15. Get your fiber. That may mean a supplemental dose each morning. Nothing is worse than not getting your fiber. Fiber cleans your pipes. You need to ingest 25-35 grams of fiber per day. Most Americans are getting maybe 1/3 of that number. It's not healthy for your body to hold onto all of that waste. Not having regular bowel movements is keeping all those toxins in your body. I struggled with potty problems for years during my starvation mode. I don't want to be gross, but I have to tell you how good it feels when you are empty.

16. Preplan your meals and have foods ready to pack in a cooler ready to go. Yeah, you are busy. I know, so am I. But if I don't preplan my meals, cook on the weekends, and cut up veggies to have ready at all times, then I can't pack my daily cooler. If I don't pack my daily cooler, than it is not convenient for me to eat healthy. Make the time for your health.

Example of Daily Food Intake (What I Would Eat)
- 1 Apple
- Chicken, tuna (in water), egg whites or egg beaters, turkey, non oily fish   [5-6x per day]
- Raw veggies or steamed: cucumbers, radishes, tomatoes, lettuce (romaine or dark leafies), asparagus, green beans, sprouts, celery, etc. Limit corn, carrots and squash. [5x per day]
- Yams and/or sweet potatoes [1 over the day]
- Oatmeal [1 cup cooked]
- Water [2-3 liters or up to half your body weight in water]
- Complex carbohydrates from fruit including: berries, grapefruit, plenty of
  [4x per day]
- 1 Piece of whole grain toast; dry [1x per day]
- Unsweetened applesauce to use as sweetener on cereal or toast [1/2 cup per day]
- Whole grain wraps [up to 2 wraps per day]
- Low fat milk [1 cup per day]
- Brown rice [1 cup cooked]
- Clear green tea, coffee and regular water
  [tea and water unlimited, coffee limit 2-4 cups]
- Unsalted nuts [A handful or half Cup]
- Nut butters (Lori likes Smart Balance Crunchy or Almond Butter

from Costco) [2 tablespoons per day]

As you can tell, you must be eating every 2-4 hours (preferably every 2-3 hours) to get your foods in! You will NEVER be hungry, which will lessen the need to binge or overeat especially during stressful days. YOU must remember to eat. Set up a reminder on your phone or PDA. Make an appointment with yourself to eat and fuel that body so it constantly burns calories. This will be the most challenging for about 2-4 weeks.

What I learned about food

Food is half the battle. It's true that working out will add to your healthy lifestyle, but if you are putting crap in your body, you will feel like crap. If you eat high fat, greasy foods, your body will store that fat and despite all your hard work at the gym, it may not appear evident.

Now, am I perfect? Absolutely not! I am alive, living in the wonderful world of great food and desserts. But I do limit myself to eating everything in a serving size. If I want a piece of cheesecake, I have a small slice. And I have to tell myself, no more of that today. Usually, if I have a party at my house, I send everyone home with care packages. I don't want to have bad stuff in my house to tempt me. It's not because I don't want to eat yummy desserts, I don't want all my hard work to go to waste. I want to be healthy for the rest of my life.

I have abused my body for years – and I will not do it anymore. I do not deserve junk food every day. As a kid, I thought I did. I'm not sure why that is; probably because my friends ate junk food and they were skinny.

Frankly, I deserve to feel good in my own skin. I deserve to have a strong healthy body. I deserve to be happy with who I am. I deserve healthy good food. I deserve to live a long healthy life.

I ate horribly for years, yo-yo dieted, and then I starved my body. My body was not happy. The abuse I did to my body is irreversible and sometimes I wonder what effects later in life I will experience. If I could go back, I would change so much, but I can't.

With all that said, you can have your favorite naughty foods from time to time, it's okay. If you deprive yourself for too long, you will want or need to binge. Just be consistent most of the time and the little "cheat meals" won't matter.

In my town of Howell, Cleary's Pub is where I go to cheat a little. Monday night is half-off pizza night and once or twice a month I go and eat some great pizza. It's okay, nothing wrong with that. I have two slices with almost every topping on it. I deserve that, too. The next day, I get right back on track and don't gain weight because of my "indiscretions" at Cleary's Pub.

Only when I am strict on myself do I find myself binging. So now I really don't do crazy strict diets. If I went according to the BMI chart in the doctor's office, I should probably be on a diet. I used to have a goal weight for myself of 127 and tried for five years through diet and exercise to attain that. One day I had the flu and lost some weight. I weighed 133, and that was the closest I ever got to 127. Sure, it's a goal but it's only a number. My doctor told me something really important and I am going to share it with you. She said, "Lori, if this is where your body has been for years, and you exercise often and eat healthy, then this is where your body wants to be. Listen to your body." I am happy with my body now and realize how right she was.

Eat healthy, exercise often and listen to your body. You don't have to be perfect. Perfection sucks. It's all our little imperfections that make us special and different from someone else.

If you eat something bad or overeat, it is just a moment in time; it does not mean your whole day is shot giving you permission to gorge yourself all day. It is just a mistake, and you need to get back on track. When it happens to me, I go and guzzle 20 ounces of water and brush, floss, and sometimes water pick my teeth. If my teeth are super clean, I usually don't want to eat anything because my teeth feel so good. Try that too, it really works.

If this is a big change for you, from your old eating habits, start slow, cutting out a bad eating habit a week, replacing it with a good eating habit. This journey is not a sprint, it's a marathon. Go slow and steady.

One final tip is my food/mood journal. I write down what I ate, what time, how much water I drank, and then how I feel. I use simple smiling faces and frowns when necessary. Graphical symbols heighten my awareness. In life we all need to be aware of our bodies. In exercise, we need to listen to our body to reduce the risk of injury. The same thing with food. I figured out by using my food/mood journal that I need to quit my complex carb intake around 3:00 p.m. I only eat carbs from fruits and veggies after 3:00 p.m. If I do eat complex carbs after that time, it gives me a stomach ache. Had I never learned this about myself, I would still have potty problems and a stomach ache almost every night.

Listen to your food/mood journal, it will tell you where the problem is and then adjust your diet until you find what works for you. My mood has greatly improved because I feel good physically.

With healthy eating and exercise you are well on your road to a happy, healthy life. You will feel better (mental), look better (physical), and your moods (emotional) will be better. A balanced physical, mental, and emotional body allows you to better enjoy your life. Take it from me, although my life is far from perfect, every day I am thankful and grateful for my life. I do not take my health for granted and I feel better than I have ever before.

You can, too.

Chapter 15
Conditions That
May Affect Your Health

At 13 or 14 years old, I was told I probably would never have children because of endometriosis. Endometriosis is a condition that is characterized by excessive growth of the lining of the uterus, called the endometrial. I began my period in 5th grade, and only had a few periods until they just stopped. It was not until my 19th birthday, I saw it again and even then it was not regular at all.

According to specialists today, endometriosis does not directly cause weight gain. I tend to disagree as I really began to put on the weight once I began my cycle and then they stopped. Other clients of mine have experienced the same weight gain. I think there is either a link of weight gain, or a link to other diseases.

Then when my daughter Torri was 7, she began to grow underarm hair. We were told all girls start puberty at different times. Other changes began too, including the weight gain. We kept Torri active and her weight in check. I knew there was a problem and began going to her pediatrician asking for help. We were told that the food she ate was partially to blame. My house had no junk food in it at all. I had already lost most of my weight and was a concerned mother. My kid went to school with a very balanced lunch box. She loved veggies, lean meats and healthy food, since she was a baby.

I remember pediatricians would still show me where Torri ranked on that dreaded BMI chart. That didn't help answer my questions. My child had a problem. I knew that and I had confirmed it. I had lived through the problem she faced and I was determined not to let her live through it, too.

Still, it took a couple of more years more years before we got her true diagnosis. Torri was diagnosed with PCOS (polycystic ovary syndrome), insulin resistance, and metabolic X. I was pretty ticked off and wanted to know more about this new diagnosis.

PCOS is a health problem that can affect a woman's menstrual cycle, ability to have children, hormones, heart, blood vessels, and appearance. With PCOS, women typically have:

- High levels of androgens, which are male hormones;
- Missed or irregular periods; and
- Many small cysts in their ovaries.

PCOS affects about 10 percent of women, according to experts. I believe it goes undiagnosed many times. The cause of PCOS is unknown. Most researchers think that more than one factor could play a role in developing PCOS. Genes are thought to be one factor. Women with PCOS tend to have a mother or sister with PCOS. Torri had me. Her symptoms were almost identical to mine. We had only slight differences.

Researchers also think insulin could be linked to PCOS. Insulin is a hormone that controls the change of sugar, starches, and other food into energy for the body to use or store. For many women with PCOS, their bodies have problems using insulin, leading to a build-up of too much insulin in the body. And this creates insulin resistance in those people. Insulin resistance makes it difficult to lose weight and increases production levels of male hormones. The male hormone is made in fat cells, ovaries, and the adrenal gland. Levels of androgen that is higher than normal can lead to excessive hair growth (not where you want it), excessive acne, weight gain, and problems with your monthly cycle.

Here are some symptoms of PCOS. But note, not all women will share the same symptoms.

- Infrequent menstrual periods, no menstrual periods, and/or irregular bleeding;
- Problems getting pregnant because you are not ovulating;
- Increased hair growth on the face, chest, stomach, back, thumbs, or toes;
- Acne, oily skin, and/or itchy scalp;
- Weight gain or obesity, usually carrying extra weight around the waist (the most unhealthy place to carry weight);
- Insulin resistance or type 2 diabetes;
- High cholesterol;

- High blood pressure;
- Male-pattern baldness or thinning hair;
- Patches of thickened and dark brown or black skin on the neck, arms, breasts, or thighs, which is actually produced by the insulin resistance;
- Skin tags, or tiny excess flaps of skin in the armpits or neck area;
- Pelvic pain;
- Anxiety or depression due to appearance and/or infertility; and
- Sleep apnea – excessive snoring and times when breathing stops while asleep.

My daughter and I shared the symptom of having no menstrual cycles. I was told I would have problems getting pregnant and Torri has been told the same. She and I both have had increased hair growth in areas we don't want hair to grow. Acne and the major weight gain happened simultaneous for both of us – at 11 for me and 13 for Torri. Although previous to the big weight gain, I was already large whereas Torri was more chubby. I had high blood pressure since 10 and Torri has been perfect with her blood pressure, even today. Pelvic pain, anxiety, depression, and skin tags were all me. Torri has sleep apnea.

There is no cure for PCOS. Doctors often mask the systems with medications not designed for this disease. I still can't believe this disease is not getting the national attention it deserves. Other diseases associated with it can lead not only to obesity, but so many other life threatening diseases. With obesity becoming one of the leading causes of death in America, this should be addressed.

Treatment of PCOS are based on a woman's symptoms, whether or not she wants to become pregnant, and lower her chances of getting heart disease and diabetes. Many women will need a combination of treatments to meet these goals.

Some treatments for PCOS include: Birth control pills which can regulate your menstrual cycles, while reducing the male hormone levels and helping with acne treatment. Progesterone can also be prescribed to control the menstrual cycle and reduce the risk of endometrial cancer.

Another treatment used is metformin (glucofage) which is used to treat type 2 diabetes. Torri was given metformin and birth control bills to try to mask her systems and enable her to have a chance to lose weight. Metaformin affects the way insulin controls blood glucose (sugar) and lowers the production of testosterone. The hair growth will begin to slow down.

Metaformin is thought to decrease body mass and improve cholesterol.

As kids, Torri and I had this thick, brown ring around our necks and inside our thighs. When I was growing up, Mom thought I didn't wash my neck. Many nights she would scrub away trying to get rid of that darn brown ring. Sometimes she put Ponds cold cream on my neck and sent me to bed, hoping what she thought was dirt would be gone by morning. It was embarrassing for me and kids at school noticed it too. I wore lots of turtlenecks and mock turtle necks to hide my neck. In the 70's and 80's it was not known readily. When I saw Torri have crazy hair growth and the brown ring, I said to myself, oh no! At age 7, we began our journey to try and figure out what it was. Torri was finally diagnosed at 14 and prescribed prescription drugs at 15.

This thick brown ring was a result of insulin resistance. It's a vicious cycle. People crave white, crappy carbs, but the more they eat, the worse their insulin resistance gets. Even though I did not know it at the time, when I dieted through starvation I only ate chicken and lettuce for years. I think ridding my body of the white, crappy carbs allowed me to lose the weight. And losing weight can put the disease in check.

Women who have PCOS usually have Metabolic Syndrome X. Metabolic Syndrome X is a grouping of cardiac risk factors that result from insulin resistance (when the body's tissues do not respond normally to insulin). A person with metabolic syndrome has a greatly increased risk of cardiovascular disease and premature death. The risk factors seen in metabolic syndrome include: insulin resistance, obesity (especially abdominal obesity), high blood pressure, abnormalities in blood clotting, and lipid abnormalities. Specifically, metabolic syndrome is diagnosed if any three of the following are present:

- Elevated waist circumference: 40 inches or more for men; 35 inches or more for women;
- Elevated triglycerides: 150 mg/dL or higher;
- Reduced HDL ("good") cholesterol: less than 40 mg/dL in men; less than 50 mg/dL in women;
- Elevated blood pressure: 130/85 mm Hg or higher; and
- Elevated fasting glucose: 100 mg/dL or higher.

Again, this Metabolic X tends to run in families and has no cure, just masking of the disease through other medicines. Although I was not diagnosed with this disease, I did meet the criteria of having four factors as a child/teen. Actually, there is one cure: to lose weight so that you are within

20 percent of your ideal weight. But it has been explained that to lose the weight with PCOS, Insulin Resistance, and Metabolic X is three-to-four times harder than an average American who does not have these diseases. That is why I call it a vicious cycle.

I believe many overweight women go undiagnosed for years and may never be diagnosed. I remember going to the doctors and having the doctor disgusted with my weight and be rude to me about it. Although I believe I added to my own problem and also gave it my all to lose the weight. Every other goal in my life I had achieved, except my weight. I had a lawn care business and lost weight every summer, but not enough to put these diseases in check. So now, I look back at all my doctors and laugh. They were partially wrong. I wasn't like the person who tries hard repeatedly and then gives us. I never gave up.

I believe that PCOS, Insulin Resistance, Metabolic X, and even Endometriosis can be controlled by losing weight. Talk to your doctor about these diseases if you have any of these symptoms. And if you have these diseases or think you have these diseases, working out with weights definitely helps. I am currently working with over 20 women with these disorders. It's not easy, but you can reduce your symptoms and lose weight. One of our clients of PT in a Box became pregnant shortly after losing a little weight and working out with weights.

If your doctor does not take you seriously and you just can't lose the weight, switch doctors. If doctors are not compassionate about helping you achieve your healthy life, dump them and try another doctor. Torri and I both have great doctors that really care about our health. In fact in April 2009, I was suddenly diagnosed with hypothyroidism and put on Armour, which is for an under active thyroid. I have had a goiter tumor on my thyroid for 15 years. Goiter, an enlargement of the thyroid gland, develops when this important metabolic gland does not have enough iodine to manufacture hormones. As it increases its cell size to try to trap more iodine, the whole gland increases in size, creating a swelling in the neck. Without supplemental iodine, a hypothyroid condition results, likely leading to fatigue and sluggishness, weight gain, and coldness of the body. At this stage, the condition may be harder to treat with iodine alone and thyroid hormone supplementation may be needed.

The Great Lakes region, i.e. Michigan, has been termed the "goiter belt" because in the 1930s, approximately 40 percent of the people in Michigan had goiter, due mainly to iodine-deficient soil. Glacier melting had washed away the iodine. The goiter on my thyroid fills up with fluid and I have the fluid removed. I just wasn't feeling my energetic self and thought something did not feel right. I took my own advice and listened to my body. Sure enough, after reading some books and researching the Internet, I had my doctor give me a blood test.

You have to be your own advocate for your own health. If you are having problems losing weight after hard work and dedication, talk to your doctor.

Other causes of weight gain:
- Stress, especially self-inflicted over losing weight;
- Oral contraceptives (women);
- Some medications, especially some anti-depressants;
- Any steroid therapy;
- Lack of sleep;
- Diabetes medications;
- High blood pressure medications;
- Heartburn medications; and
- Menopause.

You need to talk to your health care provider before stopping any medications. Talk to your doctor about suggesting another form of prescription treatment and ensure that new prescription is covered by your insurance. If you are under a lot of stress, exercise is a natural de-stressor. Exercise also helps me sleep better. Ask my husband Jeff; I am an excellent sleeper now.

The most important item is to keep a true food/mood journal. Weigh and measure your food; and keep an accurate tally of your daily intake. Then after two-four weeks, take it to your doctor. Ask for help. If your doctor does not help you, you should switch doctors.

I did use food as a crutch to deal with stress, moods, anger, any unfairness or for any reason. But had I been diagnosed earlier and there was an actual treatment, my obesity could have been curbed. I believe many of you reading this book, trying to find your healthy new life, need to take this chapter to heart. Research the Internet, talk to your doctor, be religious with your food/mood journal, and don't give up.

With all that said, work out with weights and you will see change. You will achieve your goals through proper medical care, a healthy eating plan, working out with weights, and doing your cardio. You can make the difference!

Now let's talk about Motivations!

Chapter 16
Motivations

My motivation for changing my world was a pivotal point in my life. Let's review what had transpired.

- Overweight childhood/young adulthood.
- Daughter stating to the world my favorite thing to do was "REST!"
- Taking action to change my life and my health!

I still am not perfect – there is no such thing as perfection. So don't bother trying to achieve the immeasurable, if not the impossible. I meet seemingly thin women, who complain and tell me their woes about their bodies. I used to hate these skinny women when I was overweight. I thought that they were saying the words, "I am so fat" just to get attention.

We look through magazines of celebrities and models and wish one day, we could look like them. Well, those people are airbrushed. And those people in the magazines don't lead our lives. Celebrities and models have time to devote to their bodies and hire the best personal trainers. Unless we are able to quit out jobs, I just don't think looking like a celebrity or model is an option.

Not only that, why in the world do we want to look like everyone else? Why don't we want to look like the best we can in our own bodies – the bodies that God gave us? Why can't we get to be our own best? Why can't we be happy today and set goals for our own future?

I set my goals. Life is too short and I am too busy to worry about an imperfection here or there. I have made huge improvements to how I look and feel and I really don't care what others think of me anymore – I did enough of that for most of my life.

I want the same for you. And you can do it right now. You are a great person; you deserve to be happy – and healthy. You don't have to wait any longer – and shouldn't. Start your journey today. Learn from my mistakes.

I spent my life worrying about my weight and what people thought. Guess what? People that loved me, loved me. And people that did not, did not. People that are so unhappy with their own lives made fun of me, but that is their problem and their insecurities! I chose to care about the good people in my life that love and respect me. You should, too.

So, today, at whatever your weight or goal, just be happy with who you are. And the rest will come.

This chapter is designed to help you stay on track with your goals, little things I often think about – and I want to share them with you. When you are having a bad day, pick one to lift you up.

Today is a new beginning, yesterday is gone....

You made the first step to seeing a whole new you! And I am not even talking about how you look. The WHOLE NEW YOU refers to how good you feel, how much energy you have, how confident you are, and the total well-being you enjoy. As you gain confidence in YOU, the process begins to enhance what you have – and allow the building of a stronger, healthier, and more beautiful YOU begins.

Being healthy and feeling good really "changes your world." We live in crazy times and our lives have escalated to an often too-busy lifestyle, not leaving us much time to stop and smell the roses. Or if we do have a few minutes to stop and smell the roses we are too tired to bend over to smell them. That life is no longer your life.

You will feel better and have more energy in as little as three workout sessions. I suggest everyone write a food/mood journal and remember to re-read the chapter about food and nutrition. The food/mood journal needs to be what you ate, how much, what time, how much water, coffee or other beverages you drank, and then the most important part: how your mood is at each meal or snack.

If you are like me, your mood can make you eat. I can't tell you how many pounds of potato chips, ice cream, chocolate, and Twizzlers (I love Twizzlers) I have eaten because of a bad day. Where did that get me? It got me to 242 pounds for my 5'3-1/2" frame. Why did I allow someone or something to affect me that way? Did it hurt them or improve the situation? Absolutely not.

So, (deep breath) today is the new day and you will no longer eat out of boredom, anger, sadness, or anxiety. You will eat to nourish your body so you feel good all day long. You will eat to have the energy needed to live your crazy, busy life. You will eat to feel good. This involves cutting back on high fat foods and sugary foods. You will eat to feel good about yourself and let the confidence living healthy brings into your life. It will shine through you every day. You will eat to live a long, healthy life. We are only given one body in our lifetime and we need to take care of it.

Today, you are going to begin the two week program in this book. You will complete all your workouts this week. You will stretch your muscles in between every set of weights/exercises. You will complete your cardio. And you will love yourself. You will, you will, you will.

This program was designed for you so you could look and feel your best. After each day of your workout you will begin to understand why so many people work out. Because once you do it correctly you will be hooked. Why? Because the results are unbelievable and you will have more energy, an enhanced outlook on life (elevated mood) every day you work out.

Working out with weights gives you more energy. So even if you are tired after a long day at the office, make sure you do your exercises! Do it before you sit on the couch and turn on the tube! You deserve the best. Make sure you put your health first! You can work out in the morning before the family awakens, and/or before you go to work. Or you can do it while the family members are otherwise entertained either with soccer practice, ballet, or homework. Just put yourself on the schedule and be as kind to yourself as you are to your family or co-workers.

We never have the opportunity to receive a new body – we have to re-invent the one we have. Eat healthy, exercise often, laugh continually, live your life, hang out with friends, and be happy with who you are today!

It's all about you.

It is about your goals, the size you want to be, the way you want to look, the way you want to feel, and the way you want to lead your life. Don't look through a magazine and say I want to look like her or him. Why don't you want to look like the best you? All you have to do is make the time for you, because you are worth the effort.

I was just like many of you before I got the "bug" for working out with weights. For years my husband said, "You need to weight-train. That is why you are so tired. And you could eat more food if you worked out with weights." Guess what I told him? "Honey, I have no time, I work seven days a week and have no time to add anything to my list of to-do's." I could barely find the time to sit and spend ten minutes relaxing before going to sleep at night. After all, I had to take Torri to school and cheer-leading ate up many hours, working at our antique mall (open seven days a week), planning special weekend events and promotions for our business, and finding time for siblings, parents and other relatives. I was doing so many things for other people that I never had time for myself. Remember, you can never give to others fully if you don't take the time to replenish yourself.

At my worst, I was crabby all of the time. I only ingested 300-500 calories per day, trying hard to lose the last ten pounds. Jeff was at wits end with me. He said that I was miserable, crabby, and mean. I know what you're saying to yourself, "Not Lori, she sounds so wonderful." (Ha Ha.) Well, I thought that too, until my daughter Torri stood right next to him and agreed.

They both explained that it was because I was not eating enough. This lack of food made me perpetually tired and moody. I was falling asleep as soon as I sat down at the end of my day. They were correct. They both loved me, but could not put up with my destructive methods any longer. Jeff decided that I needed motivation to weight train and purchased a membership for me and Torri at a local gym.

Dad had a brain stem stroke at 51 and shortly after he passed away. He was always thin and active but did not eat the healthiest; I wish I could have taught him what I know now.

According to Mom, when Dad gained some weight, he too had the brown ring around his neck. And actually, when Mom told me that, I remembered my Aunt Margaret too having that brown ring around her neck. And later, Aunt Margaret became seriously ill with diabetes. Insulin resistance can lead to diabetes if the risk factors are not addressed.

Life is short and you never know what's in your future, but you can change your world through fitness and healthy food choices today. Make a commitment for your health. I want you to live a long and happy life and you now have the key to ensuring that happens. Eat healthy and you can achieve anything in life. But it all takes time and attention.

Here are my favorite quotes that reinforce for me why I keep going everyday.

"Be the Change you wish to see in the world" – Gandhi

I wish to see healthy kids, teens, adults, families and older adults. I wish to see families riding their bikes together in my neighborhood after work. I wish to hear that obesity-related diseases are not killing millions of Americans. So I am going to be that change. And you can help out by spreading this message. Let's Change the World together.

"Live in the moment and make it so beautiful that it will be worth remembering." – Fanny Crosby

I am still a work in progress, but I try really try hard to live for today and make it beautiful. I especially love my job as a trainer. It's not because I like to hurt people. Although it is a good hurt. What inspires me is the look on their face, when they think they can't go on – but push themselves to greater achievements! They can and will succeed when they try. Sometimes my clients tell me they can't before they even begin an exercise and I make them do it anyway. Guess what? They can do it and then I make them do twice more than I originally wanted, just to prove my point. This applies to all of you. Today is a beautiful day, make it a memorable one. Go out and work hard, work out hard, play hard, and remember you are in control of your body and your health.

"Life isn't about finding yourself. Life is about creating yourself."
– Unknown Author

This is one of my favorites. Remember in earlier chapters, I told you my dream of losing all my excess weight and going back to my 20 year high school reunion? I thought that maybe I would be like Richard Simmons and help others lose weight. I created what I wanted. I didn't need to find myself, I knew I was a good person and smart, I just needed to create what I wanted out of my life. You can do that, too. I promise.

"Simply helping others change their world through fitness…" – Lori Wengle

That's me. I want to help you change your world. Whatever goals you set for yourself, I am here to help you. Set a goal such as this: work out three times a week. When you achieve that one goal, set another goal. Then add to the first and say, "I am going to work out three times a week and increase my reps by two on each set." And so on. Try not to set a goal about the scale, set a realistic goal such as, "I want to be in size smaller jeans by this date."
And write your action plan on how you are going to get there. Part of your action plan could be, "I am not going to eat out for a month, I am go-

ing to pack my lunch every day with healthy, attractive, good tasting foods. I will work out four days per week." If you follow through, you will be in size smaller jeans with very little effort, and in a very short time frame. Your healthy plan is all about you. You deserve this. You will succeed. Working out with weights works. Now, go change your world through fitness.

Love Yourself Today

Today is a new day, no matter what happened yesterday, each day is a new start. Remember that. Even if you have a bad day, or missed a workout, never quit. We are all a work in progress.

What does "Love Yourself Today" mean? We hear this sort of stuff over and over and yet we just won't do it or can't do it. Why? Because we are not perfect and think we don't deserve it. Get over it! You do deserve it and you are great!

Accept and love yourself as you are today – period. Love yourself for the wonderful person you are today and every day remember why you are so wonderful, because you are you and there is no one like you. In fact, list all your wonderful qualities and hang the list up on your bathroom mirror. Soon you will realize you are wonderful, and beautiful, and talented!

Does how much you weigh have anything to do with who you really are? Are you a better friend in a different size of clothing? Are you a better husband in a different size of clothes? Are you a better mechanic because of your pant size? We are the only ones that obsess about our weight or size of clothing. Does anyone else really care? We are the ones that treat ourselves differently or may not love ourselves on a particular day.

Today while writing my notes for this section a client, Lisa, called me. Lisa had fractured her ankle last week after losing a few sizes in a couple months on PT in a Box. Lisa is motivated because she sees herself melting every day and believes now that this is the program for everyone.

Lisa is upset that she has to swim for cardio, because of her ankle and does not want to. I asked, "Don't you like the water?" She replied, "I love the water." I asked, "Do you know how to do swim strokes?" Lisa said, "I know them all." I asked, "So what is the problem then?" She replied, "I don't want to wear a bathing suit. Everyone will say "look at that fat girl"."

First, no one at the pool is going to say that about Lisa. Secondly, swimming is all about Lisa. It is for Lisa, her health, and her confidence. Lisa needs to love herself and not care what others think or say. And because she is out there doing something active every day, she is loving herself.

Because of Lisa's ankle she can't do her elliptical or treadmill or bike. Lisa is so smart she talked her doctor into putting a boot on that can be taken off to swim so she can still get her cardio into her schedule and life.

I read Lisa some of what I am saying to you and it got me all riled up, because I use to be just like Lisa, even after I lost the weight. I may not have wanted to go to a beach party or even to a co-ed gym. But one day I got tired of waiting for everything in my life to be perfect and I knew I had to live my life.

Love yourself means stand up tall and do whatever you want (as long as it is legal). Live your life and don't let your weight hold you back from doing an activity, especially a healthy activity. You are who you are today and today you are wonderful.

Embrace your journey. Everything in life that is important to you requires work and your personal fitness goals are no different. This is your journey and you should embrace it and remember all your feelings each day. Maybe you can help someone else overcome their obstacles on their fitness goals.

Please love yourself, be kind to yourself, get out there and move every day, motivate others, and lead by example. You can do this. Kick your own butt every day and you will feel like a happy, healthy you.

Losing weight does not necessarily refer to a number on the scale. It's about losing fat and replacing it with lean muscle. Did you know a pound of fat at rest burns one calorie per hour, while a pound of muscle at rest burns 35 calories? You should know – I told you that fact before. You need more muscle.

A recent study looked at two women who weighed 125 pounds and who were considered "couch potatoes." The study compared them to two women who went to the gym or worked out at home four days a week and weighed 180 pounds. Guess who was fitter? The 180 pound active women that weight trained and worked out.

That is what I want for you. I want you to get healthy and find a comfortable weight that you can maintain. Take it one day at a time – and be kind to yourself. Make another change every day and keep up the good work. Pat yourself on the back daily because you deserve it.

If I want something that maybe I shouldn't have, like a special treat of some sort, it's okay to have it (but only a serving of it). If I don't eat it, I may clean out the cupboards trying to satisfy that craving. Then I'd end up eating many more calories than I would have if I would have just eaten what I wanted to begin with.

Obviously, I can't do that every day. But I do eat ice cream, cake, chips, pizza and an occasional beer (light version of course). I am a living human being that deserves some things I crave from time to time. I often go to events, after-work parties, and business luncheons where I have some of these "goodies." It's okay – really.

If you are consistent with working out, have something you want to eat from time to time. I also use my pay forward plan, which is a wonderful way to never feel guilty about what you ate. I do the extra workout first and then enjoy my treat.

We beat ourselves up enough in life. We feel guilty about a bad day, that maybe we said the wrong thing, lost our patience with our husband, or with the kids. We don't need to wreck one precious day – any day – because we ate a slice of cake. So cut it out. A serving of anything will not make you overweight. Make sure it is only a serving, and enjoy it. But the next day, work out really hard and eat healthy. Everything in moderation.

Stress, Weight & Exercise

My stressful life – or so it seemed – started when I was nine years old. I would eat because I felt family stress. I continued with that behavior for another 20 years or more until I learned to use exercise instead. But I am not alone. Stress and weight go hand-in-hand. Stressful living is at an all-time high. No wonder our waist lines match our high stress lives. So, what can we do about it?

Know this: people who exercise regularly tell you they feel better. Some will say it's because chemicals called neurotransmitters, which are produced in the brain, are stimulated during exercise. Since it's believed that neurotransmitters mediate people's moods and emotions, they can make you feel better and less stressed.

Have you ever had a really stressful day and then came home and did a strenuous job, such as cutting the grass, moving mulch, trimming bushes, or something hard? Did you feel better afterwards? Endorphins rock! Endorphins are chemicals produced naturally in the body primarily by the pituitary gland that bond to operate receptors in the nervous system like morphine or any other strong pain killer. Endorphins are also thought to be strongly linked to any sense of euphoria, and the release of sex hormones. Most people who exercise continuously have a higher concentration of endorphins resulting in "runners high." Many "exercisers" often feel they do not want to head off to the gym, but it is the "good feeling" afterwards, that keeps them going.

The euphoria and satisfaction you feel after manual labor or working out is wonderful. It's that same wonderful feeling that keeps me and my clients motivated. I use working out as a way to deal with stress. If I have a stressful day, I jump on a piece of cardio equipment. Before you know it, I feel much better.

Did you know?
- Exercise can make you eat better – People who exercise regularly tend to eat more nutritious food. And it's no secret that good nutrition helps your body manage stress better.
- Aerobic activity – All it takes is 20 minutes, six to seven days a week. Twenty minutes won't carve a big chunk out of your day, but it will significantly improve your ability to control stress.
- Recreational sports – Play tennis, racquetball, volleyball or squash. While there's no scientific evidence to conclusively support the neurotransmitter theory, there is plenty to show that exercise provides stress-relieving benefits.

There are three ways in which exercise controls stress:
- Exercise can help you feel less anxious – Exercise is being prescribed in clinical settings to help treat nervous tension. Following a session of exercise, clinicians have measured a decrease in tensed muscles. People are often less jittery and hyperactive after an exercise session.
- Exercise can relax you – One exercise session generates 90 to 120 minutes of relaxation response. Some people call this post-exercise euphoria or endorphin response. Many neurotransmitters, not just endorphins, are involved. The important thing, though, is not what they're called, but what they do: they improve your mood and leave you relaxed.
- Exercise can make you feel better about yourself – Think about those times when you've been physically active. Haven't you felt better about yourself? That feeling of accomplishment requires the kind of vigorous activity that rids your body of stress-causing adrenaline and other hormones.

If the stress is still pulling you to eat, go for a walk or run or a run/walk. Ride your bike or do something very active. Also make sure you eat six small meals a day so you are never hungry. If you think you are hungry, guzzle a 20 ounce bottle of water and brush your teeth. Wait 20 minutes. If you are still hungry have an apple or another piece of fruit. Then back to something active.

Of course, you won't be perfect every day but forgive yourself and move on. Understanding the process that I talked about today makes you aware. Awareness is another key to achieving all your goals.

Your Goals and Action Plan

Observe anyone at the top of their game and you will notice the same things. They have all had valuable guidance and direction. For personal fitness it is the same and more often than not, it comes in the form of a coach or personal trainer.

You've probably also heard the saying, if you don't like the results you are getting, than change the behavior that produced those results. So we are going to understand and develop a new strategy. Think about your top goals that you have wanted to achieve regarding your fitness. Maybe they are like these examples below.

- Look great at my high school reunion
- Drop four sizes
- Look great in a bikini
- Make your ex's jaw drop
- Run a marathon

Great, now how are you going to get these goals? If you are like me, you have tried before. But if you have never achieved those results, then let's go about this in another manner. Your goals and action plan go hand in hand. You can't achieve a goal if you don't have an action plan.

Setting small realistic goals and an action plan is all you need to achieve those goals. If you want to lose a pant size in four weeks, your action plan should consist of four-day-a-week workouts. You will want to schedule those workouts on your calendar to ensure those workouts get done.

Once you achieve that goal, then set another goal and decide on the best course of action. Again, small goals are easier to attain, and attaining your goal gives you more confidence to continue on. My goal as a kid was to be a rock star. I could sing or play an instrument, so make sure your goals are achievable.

One day, I came to my husband Jeff and showed him a cover of a magazine with my favorite fitness model Alicia Marie. I exclaimed to Jeff that I want to look just like her. Jeff said to me, "Honey, you can't look just like her." I was not very happy but I listened to him. Jeff said, "Honey, you are 38. She is in her 20s. She is 5'9-1/2" and you are 5'3-1/2". She has never been obese and you have been obese. She has brown hair and you're a blonde. She has brown eyes and yours are blue. She is African American and you're not. I hate to say it, but you are not going to look like Alicia Marie."

So, guess what I had to do? I had to find someone my age, with my body type, and set a realistic goal for myself. If you can never achieve your goals then you will not stick to your new healthy lifestyle. Just be realistic. In my case, I had to embrace my body and make it the best I could for me. I am not in my 20's, which is good for me, because I have never looked better!

The moral to the story is to set realistic goals and smaller ones. You can add to your goals and your action plan as you go. Your goal might be to lose a pant size and your action plan will include working out four days a week – and only go out to dinner one day a week. In a month, when you achieve that goal, set a new goal and a new action plan to accomplish that goal. Be realistic and kind to yourself and you will achieve all your goals and will look and feel great!

No More Excuses

Become aware of your excuses, implement a different way of thinking, and live in the now (no more I wishes). Stop saying you will change tomorrow. Do it today. If you want to see change in your body, be willing to do the work and have passion to do the work and compassion for yourself.

Pack your gym bag and go straight from work. Whether you go to a gym or a local park.

Prepare your food for the week on Sundays. Cook a few meals ahead of time and grill up chicken breast to ensure you have food handy to grab and pack a nutritious lunch. Prepare healthy dinners and have them ready to pop into the oven – and then go take the dog for a speedy walk while your dinner is cooking. If you don't have a dog, take yourself for a speedy walk.

Buy a veggie tray every week to ensure you have healthy snacks. Have hummus or low calorie dips to compliment your fresh veggies.

Have a plan for a bad day. Have ten fun, healthy things to do to change your day around if something wrong happens. If you faltered on your healthy eating goals or skipped a workout session, have a makeup plan to reinforce the new you.

Implement the "Pay Forward Plan" to help you rid your life of guilt when you are tempted at a dinner, wedding, or activity that you may indulge.

The Pay Forward Plan

This is what I do so that I can never make up excuses of why I miss a workout or eat something I shouldn't have. I call it the Pay Forward Plan.

If I know I may be tempted with something I really like. When that happens, I do a few minutes per day of extra cardio to save up my burned calories for something good I want to eat. To get your yummy treat, you must have banked the extra calories before you indulge in the treat. It's hard to do the workout after you have enjoyed the treat.

If I am going to a wedding and want to enjoy the dinner, dessert, and a couple glasses of wine, than I just do 5-10 extra minutes of cardio a few days in the week prior. I save up the calories I burned and then the feeling of guilt does not bother me. I already earned my treat.

The same holds true for my cardio and workouts. I do extra cardio and save up my minutes to skip a day, or do extra weight training on days that I get done quicker. I add some of my exercises from the next day's workout and when I am done with all my exercises I am really done for the week.

Whatever excuses you have, make the time for your new healthy lifestyle. You deserve this new you, so remember that and continue on with the journey to the new you. Your body will thank you in the future. You will be stronger, have more energy, feel and look confident, and finally feel good in your skin. Your goals will be attained and maintained through working out with weights.

Lifting Heavy Weights

The five keys to working out effectively are muscle confusion, heavy weights, consistency, stretching, and cardio. And you can't train like a girl, even if you are a girl. Huh? Let me explain.

You need to switch up your routine continually. Every week a different set of exercises. It should take about three-five weeks to repeat an exercise for best results. This causes muscle confusion, the key to any result driven workout. If you want to see continual results you must continually switch up your routine. The exercise you pick for week one you should not repeat for weeks. I don't care if you don't like the one of the exercises. Just do it and you will learn to like it.

Have you ever bought exercise merchandise you saw on a TV ad? Did it work for you all of the time? Probably not and so you quit. That is exactly what happened to me. I would do something and see results, but then the results would slow or stop and I would become discouraged. When step aerobics first came out I bought one of the "Buns of Steel" and it worked. I felt the pain. But I kept doing the same routine over and over and I stopped seeing results as quickly. I grew bored and so did my muscles. Once the results were not consistent, I quit. I could name a hundred other programs that I have tried.

It was not until I hired a personal trainer that I realized that by not doing the same thing over and over again, I was able to see positive results. It was a "Eureka!" moment for me. Then I wanted to learn more, so I bought some fitness magazines and learned more exercises and read about why. I needed to know why and the trainer I had couldn't tell me. It's called muscle confusion, something I have mentioned before in this book. The main principle is to confuse the body by eliminating the muscle plateau that is common among all workout regiments.

I refer to it as switching it up, constantly picking new exercises for each muscle group. In three-five weeks you can repeat the exercise and your muscles don't remember. Each exercise may just be a little different than the previous week and may use different hand position. An example is the Triceps Dip, where, using a bench or your couch, you hold yourself straight up and then dip down until your butt slightly touches the floor. Another exercise, Triceps Rope Pull down is where you have a rope handle on a high pulley and you keep your elbows close to your sides as you pull the rope down and out. Each of these two triceps exercises hit your triceps differently. There are three heads to a triceps muscle and some exercises may work two of the three heads and some may work a different one.

How heavy do I go with my weights? The key is to lift heavy enough weights that your last two reps of each set are very hard to complete. Have you ever been to a gym and noticed that there is spit all over the mirror? Not a pleasant sight. I did and I thought to myself, who the heck is spitting on the mirrors? Well now I know. Everyone really pushes hard to see results. Sometimes my clients say, "I can't do that weight or that machine." I prove them wrong every time. They do it – and then they do more.

If you really want to see unbelievable results, then lift heavy weights. Why? Because if you replace fat with lean muscle, your metabolism will increase for up to 48 hours which means you will be a fat burning machine after a workout, even while you are sitting on the couch watching TV.

I had a client that refused to change her eating habits so I kicked her butt three times a week for six months and she lost 34 pounds. (Actually she gave up her one vice, too – Goober Grape.) This is a true story but it is not the way to be healthy forever. You need to balance your food, exercise, and relaxation all together. That client is now eating very healthy and feels better. On top of that, her digestion is great and her skin is clear.

Consistency is another key. You need to work out with weights each muscle group every week. A three-day program is perfect for beginners. Once you achieved your goal, you could train as little as twice a week and maintain.

You should still need to do your cardio, three-six times a week. Cardio is muscle training for your heart and lungs. Cardio helps your heart and lungs continue to stay strong and work the way they are suppose to work. Even a "higher authority" would agree.

The U.S. Surgeon General recommends that everyone do moderate exercise six days a week. I agree, but there are many forms that you can fit this into your schedule. Join an adult baseball, basketball, flag football, hockey, or tennis league. If you can't find one, start one. Go to a metro park and bring your bike, rollerblades, or walking poles. You can fit a couple hours of cardio into your schedule because you will feel so good.

And finally, start stretching. Make sure you stretch each muscle group in between each of your sets of exercises. And then once warmed up on cardio, take another moment to stretch. Never stretch a cold muscle. Always do 5-10 minutes of cardio before beginning. If you stretch between sets, this will create long, lean muscles. Flexibility is key and as we get older, we lose our flexibility. Guys, you need to stretch too. It will help you stay limber and create larger muscles. Girls, we can't get huge muscles without steroids. It will create longer lines and help reduce the risk of injury.

So now get out there and confuse your muscles by switching up your routine, lift heavy weights, be consistent, do cardio three-six times per week and stretch in between your sets. You will be on the road to a new you!

Fat Loss and You

I understand how hard it is to diet and continue to stay on track. That's why I failed for years. I would get bigger every time I went on a diet. I would achieve my skinny of 180 pounds. At 180 pounds I felt great and looked attractive. I cut 65 lawns per week every summer and would get down to 180 pounds usually every summer.

The manual labor (those were the days of push lawn mowers) really added muscle to my frame and I melted the weight off out in the sun and heat while doing some hard work. I just could not maintain that loss until I discovered weight training. Once I saw the continual results of weight training and saw my problems areas improve I continued on. Then my curiosity of why and how weight training worked kicked into overdrive and I began to read everything I could. I soon discovered why weight training worked so well. Here it is – again: One pound of muscle at rest burns 35 calories per day, while one pound of fat burns only one calorie.

Here is an example of switching out five pounds of fat for five pounds of muscle. (Your results may vary depending on starting weight and current muscle.)

Muscle
35 Calories per Day X 5 pounds = 175 X 365 days =63,775
One pound equals 3,500 calories
63,775 divided by 3500=18.2
Fat
1 Calorie per day X 5 pounds = 5 X 365 = 1,825
One pound equals 3500 calories

So without dieting, changing five pounds of fat into five pounds of muscle will melt your body by 18.2 pounds in a year – without changing your diet. Now, for hundreds of other reasons, you need to eat healthy and eat more often. But this explanation should show you how this will continue to work for you forever.

When we weight train we burn fat for 48 hours to 72 hours. So if you work out with weights every other day, you will continually burn fat. Your metabolism will increase and the food that you do eat will burn as fuel that your body needs to workout.

I can't say this enough: If you work out with weights, you will see your body melt. If you change your eating bad habits and eat five-six times a day, include healthy choices such as complex carbs, lean protein, fruits and veggies, as well as dairy and good oils, you will see the most fantastic results.

I don't believe any of us are lazy or don't want to achieve our goals for our weight. If you were, you wouldn't be reading this book. I firmly believe some programs out there that are not attainable, do not work, involve too much time or money, or don't interest us. If something really works, you will see continual results – and you will continue.

Working out with weights will add unbelievable energy to your life. If you are thinking you do not have the time to work out, think again. You should work out for the constant energy it provides. Working out with weights can help with stress, moods, pregnancy, post pregnancy moods and body image, your sex life for men and women, muscular strength, flexibility, stability, and balance.

Just three days a week and you will be hooked. You will see your body melt and feel and look your best. It's not about the number on the scale; you will know when you achieve your goal. You will feel good in your own skin. You will be confident and full of energy. You will be the best you can be. And then you will be telling everyone you know to work out with weights.

So get out there and do it and Change Your World!

Alarming Statistics & Breaking the Cycle

This is the first time in American history that our kids will not live as long as we will and this is due to obesity related diseases. Let me explain, so this really sinks in.

Our children will die at an age younger than we will. For example, women are averaging a 75-year lifespan and our children will not live that long, reversing an upward trend we have seen for decades. Are you kidding me? How can this happen with all of the medical advances and "miracle drugs" we have experienced?

We are leading such busy lives, working longer hours, commuting more hours per week and running ourselves ragged. We don't make the time to exercise, be active, and keep our kids active enough. Our busy lives cause us to eat on the run and eat prepared foods.

We all need to go back to the basics. Exercise more, be active, lead by example and eat at home, pack our lunches and break this cycle.

Here are more statistics I want your help to change. Statistics sometimes are hard to listen to, so please listen to this, it will change your world. Obesity is a major risk factor for coronary heart disease, high blood pressure, stroke, diabetes, and some forms of cancer. Obese people are also at high risk for depression, job discrimination, and other social problems. Some 300,000 premature deaths are caused by obesity each year. About $100 billion in annual health care costs are attributed to obesity. After tobacco use, obesity is the second leading cause of preventable deaths. Can you imagine, obesity is just behind cigarettes.

About six out of 10 Americans are overweight or obese, and those numbers are rising. The number of children and teens who are overweight or obese is also rising. If anyone goes into the school systems today, over-weight kids are about half of the student population.

According to the United States Surgeon General Richard H. Carmona, "[Poor] health affects every state, every city, every community, and every school across our great nation. The crisis is obesity. It's the fastest-growing cause of disease and death in America. And it's completely preventable. One out of every eight deaths in America is caused by an illness directly related to overweight and obesity".

It has been estimated that the annual cost of being overweight and obese in the U.S. is $122.9 billion. This estimate accounts for $64.1 billion in direct costs and $58.8 billion in indirect costs related to the obesity epi-demic, a sum that is comparable to the economic costs of cigarette smok-ing. Direct health care costs for obesity refer to preventive, diagnostic, and treatment services (e.g., physician visits, medications, and hospital and nursing home care) for obesity-related diseases and conditions (heart disease, hypertension, diabetes); while indirect costs related to the obesity epidemic are the value of wages lost by people unable to work because of illness or disability, as well as the value of future earnings lost by prema-ture death. Obesity and obesity-related conditions or ailments result in at least $62.7 million in doctors' visits and $39.3 million in lost workdays each year .

Obesity Demographics
- Obesity is the second leading cause of preventable death in the U.S.
- Approximately 127 million adults in the U.S. are overweight, 60 million are obese (Body Mass Index or BMI > 30) and 9 million are extremely obese (Body Mass Index or BMI > 40) .
- Currently, an estimated 65.2 percent of U.S. adults, age 20 years and older, and 15 percent of children and adolescents are over-weight and 30.5 percent are obese (childhood or pediatric obe-sity).
- Approximately 62 percent of female Americans are considered overweight.
- Approximately 67 percent of male Americans are considered over-weight.

- An estimated 400,000 deaths per year may be attributable to poor diet and low physical activity.
- It is estimated that 25-70 percent of the difference in weight between individuals is hereditary or genetic. However, it is important to remember that genetic predisposition only impacts an individual's tendency towards obesity.
- Researchers at the U.S. Centers for Disease Control and Prevention (CDC) estimated that as many as 47 million Americans may exhibit a cluster of medical conditions (a "metabolic syndrome" or "Syndrome X") characterized by insulin resistance and the presence of obesity, excessive abdominal fat, high blood sugar and triglycerides, high blood pressure (hypertension) and high cholesterol .

Other Factors for Success in Helping Americans Change Their World

Currently, The American Council on Exercise (A.C.E) has lobbied congress to allow Personal Spending Accounts, typically used for medical procedures or products, such as glasses or selective surgeries to be used for gym memberships and personal trainers. This is needed to help the costs of getting fit especially in today's world.

Corporate America Incents Employees to Get Fit

Corporate America is trying to reduce health care costs through incentives for employees to get healthy. All you have to do is read or listen to the national news and you will see and hear about these incentive packages. Some companies are even going as far as to charge employees weekly or monthly fees to help cover rising health care costs for such things as being overweight, smoking, high cholesterol. These employees can deter these charges by enrolling in weight watchers, start a stop smoking program or other programs offered and paid for by the employer.

Counting the Cost of Poor Fitness in the Workplace

Check out these statistics:
1. American industry loses $32 billion and 132 million workdays are lost every year because of employee's premature deaths that are associated with cardiovascular disease (high blood pressure, heart stroke, diabetes, and obesity.) Billions more are lost as a result of lowered productivity as a result of sickness and disability.
2. The National Safety Council stated that in 1996 backaches alone

cost industry over $1.2 billion in production and services, and $275 million more in worker's compensation. Corporate fitness and wellness concepts have become a management tool for many industries, including Johnson & Johnson, Xerox, and General Motors are a few examples of companies that incorporate fitness in the workplace.

3. For every dollar a company spends on back surgery, they'll spend three to five times that amount on indirect costs such as productive loss, rehiring, retraining, and overtime.

4. Approximately $14 billion is spent annually on medical care and absenteeism directly related to back pain.

5. More than 60% of all reported workplace illnesses are attributed to repetitive strain disorders caused by improper or overuse of the hand and arm muscles. In 1992 alone, there were nearly 90,000 people in private industry who missed work, often six weeks or more, because of repetitive motion injuries.

6. There are an estimated 45 million Americans who suffer from chronic headaches. They make more than 50 million office visits a year to doctors and spend more than $400 million on over the counter pain relievers. Industry loses at least $55 million a year due to absenteeism and medical expenses caused by headaches.

7. The average employer spends more than $8,000 per year for each employee's health benefits, including insurance, disability and worker's compensation.

8. According to a three-year study by Motorola comparing costs for employees that participated in its wellness initiatives compared to those that didn't, for every $1 the company invested in wellness benefits, it saved $3.93.

9. Johnson & Johnson reported that their employee's had taken 13% fewer sick days the first year of their involvement in an organized exercise program and even fewer sick days by the second year. Other studies have found similar decreases in absenteeism either in the company as a whole or in program participants after the introduction of a fitness program. Absenteeism alone can cause loss of production of about 6 days per worker per year in non-union operations and 10-14 days per worker in union operations.

With all that said, I still cringe at the first statistic I spoke of, allowing our children to certainly live as long as we do. Our children should live as long or longer than we do! We need to lead by example, we can change the world!

We can **CHANGE YOUR WORLD**.

Image Captions